ODE/PDE Analysis
of Multiple Myeloma

ODE/PDE Analysis of Multiple Myeloma

Programming in R

William E. Schiesser

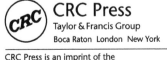

CRC Press
Taylor & Francis Group
Boca Raton London New York

CRC Press is an imprint of the
Taylor & Francis Group, an **informa** business

Library of Congress Cataloging-in-Publication Data

Names: Schiesser, W. E., author.
Title: ODE/PDE analysis of multiple myeloma : programming in R / William E. Schiesser.
Description: First edition. | Boca Raton, FL : CRC Press, 2020. | Includes bibliographical references and index. | Summary: "The intent of this book is to present a methodology for the formulation and computer implementation of mathematical models for multiple myeloma, a form of bone cancer. The models are stated as systems of ordinary and partial differential equations (ODE/PDEs). The ODE/PDE methodology is presented through a series of examples, starting with a basic ODE model in chapter 1, and concluding with a detailed ODE/PDE model in chapter 4 that gives the spatiotemporal distribution of four components in the bone marrow and peripheral blood. The computer-based implementation of the example models is presented through routines coded (programmed) in R, a quality, open-source scientific computing system that is readily available from the Internet. Formal mathematics is minimized, e.g., no theorems and proofs. Rather, the presentation is through detailed examples that the reader/researcher/analyst can execute on modest computers. The PDE analysis is based on the method of lines (MOL), an established general algorithm for PDEs, implemented with finite differences. The routines are available from a download link so that the example models can be executed without having to first study numerical methods and computer coding. The routines can then be applied to variations and extensions of the multiple myeloma models, such as changes in the ODE/PDE parameters (constants) and form of the model equations."-- Provided by publisher.
Identifiers: LCCN 2020000933 | ISBN 9780367471354 (hardback) | ISBN 9780367473549 (ebook)
Subjects: LCSH: Multiple myeloma--Mathematical models. | Numerical analysis--Computer programs. | R (Computer program language)
Classification: LCC RC280.B6 S34 2020 | DDC 616.99/418--dc23
LC record available at https://lccn.loc.gov/2020000933

ISBN: 978-0-367-47135-4 (hbk)
ISBN: 978-0-367-49551-0 (pbk)
ISBN: 978-0-367-47354-9 (ebk)

Typeset in Times
by Lumina Datamatics Limited

Visit the companion website: https://www.lehigh.edu/~wes1/dpde_download/
Visit the e-Resources: https://routledge.com/9780367471354

To Anne Drennan and Gary Kohler,
with deep appreciation for your support.

Contents

Preface

Multiple myeloma is a cancer of the bone marrow plasma cells. Normal plasma cells are an important part of the immune system.

Mathematical models for multiple myeloma based on ordinary and partial differential equations (ODE/PDEs) are presented in this book, starting with a basic ODE model in Chapter 1, and concluding with a detailed ODE/PDE model in Chapters 4 and 5 that gives the spatiotemporal distribution of four dependent variable components in the bone marrow and peripheral blood: (1) protein produced by multiple myeloma cells, termed the M protein, (2) cytotoxic T lymphocytes ($CTLs$), (3) natural killer (NK) cells, and (4) regulatory T cells (T_{regs}).

The computer-based implementation of the example models is presented through routines coded (programmed) in R, a quality, open-source scientific computing system that is readily available from the Internet. Formal mathematics is minimized, e.g., no theorems and proofs. Rather, the presentation is through detailed examples that the reader/researcher/analyst can execute on modest computers. The PDE analysis is based on the method of lines (MOL), an established general algorithm for PDEs, implemented with finite differences.

The routines are available from a download link (https://www.routledge.com/9780367471354) so that the example models can be executed without having to first study numerical methods and computer coding. The routines can then be applied to variations and extensions of the multiple myeloma models, such as changes in the ODE/PDE parameters (constants) and form of the model equations.

The author would welcome comments/suggestions concerning this approach to multiple myeloma analysis (directed to wes1@lehigh.edu).

William E. Schiesser
Bethlehem, PA

Author

William E. Schiesser is the Emeritus McCann Professor in the chemical and biomolecular engineering department at Lehigh University as well as a former professor in the mathematics department. He recently authored several books on computer-based solutions to model real-life phenomena, such as the development of Parkinson's disease. He holds a PhD from Princeton University and an honorary ScD from the University of Mons, Belgium. He is the author or co-author of a series of books in his field of research on numerical methods and associated software for ordinary, differential-algebraic and partial differential equations (ODE/DAE/PDEs) and the development of mathematical models based on ODE/DAE/PDEs.

1 Introductory ODE Model

(1) Introduction

The following background statement from [1] defines the term *multiple myeloma*:

> Multiple myeloma is a cancer of plasma cells. Normal plasma cells are found in the bone marrow and are an important part of the immune system. The immune system is made up of several types of cells that work together to fight infections and other diseases. Lymphocytes (lymph cells) are one of the main types of white blood cells in the immune system and include T cells and B cells. Lymphocytes are in many areas of the body, such as lymph nodes, the bone marrow, the intestines, and the bloodstream.
>
> When B cells respond to an infection, they mature and change into plasma cells. Plasma cells make the antibodies (also called immunoglobulins) that help the body attack and kill germs. Plasma cells, are found mainly in the bone marrow. Bone marrow is the soft tissue inside bones. In addition to plasma cells, normal bone marrow is also the home for other blood cells such as red cells, white cells, and platelets.
>
> In general, when plasma cells become cancerous and grow out of control, this is called multiple myeloma. The plasma cells make an abnormal protein (antibody) known by several different names, including monoclonal immunoglobulin, monoclonal protein (M-protein), M-spike, or paraprotein.

As further background, multiple myeloma (MM) is a cancer of plasma blood cells [1]. The MM model discussed initially in Chapter 1 [1,2] defines as a function of time the concentrations in the blood stream of: (1) protein produced by MM cells, termed the M protein, (2) cytotoxic T lymphocytes ($CTLs$), (3) natural killer (NK) cells, and (4) regulatory T cells (T_{regs}). CTLs, NK cells, and T_{regs} are the immune system's response to the MM cells.

The initial model consists of four ordinary differential equations (ODEs). The solution to the ODEs is computed with a library routine for initial value ODEs available in R[1]. The R routines that implement the model are next listed and discussed in detail.

The routines are also available through a download link so that the reader/analyst/researcher can access them to confirm the reported solutions. The routines can then be modified and extended for computer-based experimentation with the model.

The ODE model is extended to a system of partial differential equations (PDEs) in subsequent chapters to define the spatiotemporal distribution of (1)–(4) in the bone marrow where the cancer originates, and in the peripheral blood.

(1.1)   ODE model

The 4×4 (four ODEs in four unknowns) model is stated as eqs. (1.1).

$$\frac{dM}{dt} = s_M + r_M \left(1 - \frac{M}{K_M}\right) M$$

$$-\delta_M \left[1 + \left(\frac{a_{NM}N}{b_{NM} + N} + \frac{a_{CM}T_C}{b_{CM} + T_C} + a_{CNM} \frac{N}{b_{NM} + N} \cdot \frac{T_C}{b_{CM} + T_C}\right) \cdot \right.$$

$$\left. \left(1 - \frac{a_{MM}M}{b_{MM} + M} - \frac{a_{RM}T_R}{b_{RM} + T_R}\right)\right] \cdot M \qquad (1.1\text{-}1)$$

$$\frac{dT_C}{dt} = r_C \left(1 - \frac{T_C}{K_C}\right) \left(1 + \frac{a_{MC}M}{b_{MC} + M} + \frac{a_{NC}N}{b_{NC} + N}\right) T_C - \delta_C T_C \qquad (1.1\text{-}2)$$

$$\frac{dN}{dt} = s_N + r_N \left(1 - \frac{N}{K_N}\right) \left(1 + \frac{a_{CN}T_C}{b_{CN} + T_C}\right) N - \delta_N N \qquad (1.1\text{-}3)$$

$$\frac{dT_R}{dt} = r_R \left(1 - \frac{T_R}{K_R}\right) \left(1 + \frac{a_{MR}M}{b_{MR} + M}\right) T_R - \delta_R T_R \qquad (1.1\text{-}4)$$

---

[1] R is a quality open source scientific computing system that is available from the Internet [4].

The dependent variables of eqs. (1.1) are listed in Table 1.1.

Table 1.1: Dependent variables of eqs. (1.1)

$M(t)$	protein produced by MM cells
$T_C(t)$	cytotoxic T lymphocytes ($CTLs$)
$N(t)$	natural killer (NK) cells
$T_R(t)$	regulatory T cells (T_{regs})

A schematic diagram of eqs. (1.1) is given in [2], Figure 1.

Equations (1.1) are first order in t, so each requires one initial condition (IC).

$$M(t = 0) = M^0 = 4 \qquad (1.2\text{-}1)$$

$$T_C(t = 0) = T_C^0 = 464 \qquad (1.2\text{-}2)$$

$$N(t = 0) = N^0 = 227 \qquad (1.2\text{-}3)$$

$$T_R(t = 0) = T_R^0 = 42 \qquad (1.2\text{-}4)$$

The initial values, $4, 464, 227, 42$, are taken from [2], Table 2.

The parameters in eqs. (1.1) are taken from [2], base case of Table 2.

Table 1.2: Parameters of eqs. (1.1)

Eq. (1.1-1)		
$s_M = 0.001$	$r_M = 0.0175$	$K_M = 10$
$\delta_M = 0.002$	$a_{NM} = 5$	$b_{NM} = 150$
$a_{CM} = 5$	$b_{CM} = 375$	$a_{CNM} = 8$
$a_{MM} = 0.5$	$b_{MM} = 3$	$a_{RM} = 0.5$
$b_{RM} = 25$		
Eq. (1.1-2)		
$r_C = 0.013$	$K_C = 800$	$a_{MC} = 5$
$b_{MC} = 3$	$a_{NC} = 1$	$b_{NC} = 150$
$\delta_C = 0.02$		
Eq. (1.1-3)		
$s_N = 0.03$	$r_N = 0.04$	$K_N = 450$
$a_{CN} = 1$	$b_{CN} = 375$	$\delta_N = 0.025$
Eq. (1.1-4)		
$r_R = 0.0831$	$K_R = 80$	$a_{MR} = 2$
$b_{MR} = 3$	$\delta_R = 0.0757$	

The nonlinear interaction terms of eqs. (1.1) are explained briefly in Table 1.3 as in [2], Table 1.

Table 1.3: Brief explanation of the interaction terms of eqs. (1.1)

Term	Equation	Interaction
$\left(\dfrac{a_{NM}N}{b_{NM}+N}\right)M$	(1.1-1)	N cells kill myeloma cells and decrease M
$\left(\dfrac{a_{CM}T_C}{b_{CM}+T_C}\right)M$	(1.1-1)	T_C cells kill myeloma cells and decrease M
$\left(a_{CNM}\dfrac{N}{b_{NM}+N}\cdot\dfrac{T_C}{b_{CM}+T_C}\right)M$	(1.1-1)	T_C increases activation/efficacy of N
$\left(\dfrac{a_{MM}M}{b_{MM}+M}\right)$	(1.1-1)	Myeloma cells decrease efficacy of N and T_C
$\left(\dfrac{a_{RM}T_R}{b_{RM}+T_R}\right)$	(1.1-1)	T_R decreases efficacy of N and T_C
$\left(\dfrac{a_{MC}M}{b_{MC}+M}\right)T_C$	(1.1-2)	Antigens shed from M stimulate T_C proliferation
$\left(\dfrac{a_{NC}N}{b_{NC}+N}\right)T_C$	(1.1-2)	N crosstalk with T_C; boosts T_C proliferation
$\left(\dfrac{a_{CN}T_C}{b_{CN}+T_C}\right)N$	(1.1-3)	T_C crosstalk with N; boosts N proliferation
$\left(\dfrac{a_{MR}M}{b_{MR}+M}\right)T_R$	(1.1-4)	Myeloma cells boost T_R proliferation

The parameters (constants) in Table 1.3 have the numerical values in Table 1.2.

Equations (1.1), (1.2) constitute the ODE model which are integrated (solved) numerically with a library initial value ODE integrator, `lsodes` [4]. The R routines that implement the integration are considered next, starting with a main program.

(1.1.1)   Main program for the ODE model

The main program for eqs. (1.1), (1.2) is in Listing 1.1.

Listing 1.1: Main program for eqs. (1.1), (1.2)

```
#
#   Four ODE MM model
#
# Delete previous workspaces
  rm(list=ls(all=TRUE))
```

(Continued)

```
  Listing 1.1 (Continued): Main program for eqs. (1.1), (1.2)

#
# Access ODE integrator
  library("deSolve");
#
# Access functions for numerical solution
  setwd("f:/multipleMyeloma/chap1");
  source("ode1a.R");
#
# Parameters
#
# Eq. (1.1-1)
  sM = 0.001; rM = 0.0175; KM = 10;
  delM = 0.002; aNM = 5; bNM = 150;
  aCM = 5; bCM = 375; aCNM = 8;
  aMM = 0.5; bMM = 3; aRM = 0.5;
  bRM = 25;
#
# Eq. (1.1-2)
  rC =0.013; KC = 800; aMC = 5;
  bMC = 3; aNC = 1; bNC = 150;
  delC = 0.02;
#
# Eq. (1.1-3)
  sN = 0.03; rN = 0.04; KN = 450;
  aCN = 1; bCN= 375; delN = 0.025;
#
# Eq. (1.1-4)
  rR = 0.0831; KR = 80; aMR = 2;
  bMR = 3; delR = 0.0757;
#
# Independent variable for ODE integration
  t0=0;tf=1.0e+03;nout=41;
  tout=seq(from=t0,to=tf,by=(tf-t0)/(nout-1));
#
# Initial conditions (t=0)
  y0=rep(0,4);
  y0[1]=4;
  y0[2]=464;
```

(Continued)

Listing 1.1 (Continued): Main program for eqs. (1.1), (1.2)

```
y0[3]=227;
y0[4]=42;
ncall=0;
#
# ODE integration
out=lsodes(y=y0,times=tout,func=ode1a,
    sparsetype ="sparseint",rtol=1e-6,
    atol=1e-6,maxord=5);
nrow(out)
ncol(out)
#
# Arrays for plotting numerical solution
 M=rep(0,nout);
TC=rep(0,nout);
 N=rep(0,nout);
TR=rep(0,nout);
for(it in 1:nout){
   M[it]=out[it,2];
  TC[it]=out[it,3];
   N[it]=out[it,4];
  TR[it]=out[it,5];
}
#
# Display numerical solution
cat(sprintf("\n           t       M(t)       TC(t)
            N(t)       TR(t)"));
iv=seq(from=1,to=nout,by=2);
for(it in iv){
  cat(sprintf("%10.2f %10.3f %10.3f %10.3f %10.3f\n",
             tout[it],M[it],TC[it],N[it],TR[it]));
}
#
# Calls to ODE routine
cat(sprintf("\n\n ncall = %5d\n\n",ncall));
#
# Plot ODE solutions
#
# M(t)
 plot(tout,M,xlab="time (days)",ylab="M(t)",
   xlim=c(t0,tf),main="",type="l",lwd=2,
   col="black");
```

(Continued)

```
  Listing 1.1 (Continued): Main program for eqs. (1.1), (1.2)

#
# TC(t)
  plot(tout,TC,xlab="time (days)",ylab="TC(t)",
    xlim=c(t0,tf),main="",type="l",lwd=2,
    col="black");
#
# N(t)
  plot(tout,N,xlab="time (days)",ylab="N(t)",
    xlim=c(t0,tf),main="",type="l",lwd=2,
    col="black");
#
# TR(t)
  plot(tout,TR,xlab="time (days)",ylab="TR(t)",
    xlim=c(t0,tf),main="",type="l",lwd=2,
    col="black");
```

We can note the following details about the main program of Listing 1.1.

- Previous workspaces are deleted.

```
#
#   Four ODE MM model
#
# Delete previous workspaces
  rm(list=ls(all=TRUE))
```

- The R ODE integrator library deSolve is accessed. Then the directory with the files for the solution of eqs. (1.1), (1.2) is designated. Note that setwd (set working directory) uses / rather than the usual \.

```
#
# Access ODE integrator
  library("deSolve");
#
# Access functions for numerical solution
  setwd("f:/multipleMyeloma/chap1");
  source("ode1a.R");
```

ode1a.R is the routine with the programming of eqs. (1.1), (1.2).

- The model parameters are specified numerically.

```
#
# Parameters
#
# Eq. (1.1-1)
  sM = 0.001; rM = 0.0175; KM = 10;
  delM = 0.002; aNM = 5; bNM = 150;
  aCM = 5; bCM = 375; aCNM = 8;
  aMM = 0.5; bMM = 3; aRM = 0.5;
  bRM = 25;
#
# Eq. (1.1-2)
  rC =0.013; KC = 800; aMC = 5;
  bMC = 3; aNC = 1; bNC = 150;
  delC = 0.02;
#
# Eq. (1.1-3)
  sN = 0.03; rN = 0.04; KN = 450;
  aCN = 1; bCN= 375; delN = 0.025;
#
# Eq. (1.1-4)
  rR = 0.0831; KR = 80; aMR = 2;
  bMR = 3; delR = 0.0757;
```

- An interval in t of 41 points is defined for $0 \leq t \leq 1000$ so that tout=0,1000/40,...,1000.

```
#
# Independent variable for ODE integration
  t0=0;tf=1.0e+03;nout=41;
  tout=seq(from=t0,to=tf,by=(tf-t0)/(nout-1));
```

- ICs (1.2) are defined (from [1]).

```
#
# Initial conditions (t=0)
  y0=rep(0,4);
  y0[1]=4;
  y0[2]=464;
  y0[3]=227;
  y0[4]=42;
  ncall=0;
```

Also, the counter for the calls to **ode1a** is initialized.

- The system of 4 ODEs is integrated by the library integrator lsodes (available in deSolve, [4]). As expected, the inputs to lsodes are the ODE function, ode1a, the IC vector y0, and the vector of output values of t, tout. The length of y0 (4) informs lsodes how many ODEs are to be integrated. func,y,times are reserved names.

```
#
# ODE integration
  out=lsodes(y=y0,times=tout,func=ode1a,
      sparsetype ="sparseint",rtol=1e-6,
      atol=1e-6,maxord=5);
  nrow(out)
  ncol(out)
```

The numerical solution to the ODEs is returned in matrix out. In this case, out has the dimensions $nout \times (4 + 1) = 41 \times 5$, which are confirmed by the output from nrow(out),ncol(out) (included in the numerical output considered subsequently). The offset $+1$ is required since the first element of out is the value of t, and the 2 to 5 elements are the values of $M(t), T_C(t), N(t), T_R(t)$.

- Vectors are defined for the computed ODE solution (in array out returned by lsodes). The solution is then placed in these arrays.

```
#
# Arrays for plotting numerical solution
  M=rep(0,nout);
  TC=rep(0,nout);
  N=rep(0,nout);
  TR=rep(0,nout);
  for(it in 1:nout){
    M[it]=out[it,2];
    TC[it]=out[it,3];
    N[it]=out[it,4];
    TR[it]=out[it,5];
  }
```

Again, the offset +1 is required since the first element of each solution vector (for a particular index it) is the value of t associated with the solution.

- The four dependent variables $M(t), T_C(t), N(t), T_R(t)$ are displayed as a function of t with a for. Every second value of t appears from by=2.

```
#
# Display numerical solution
```

```
    cat(sprintf("\n                 t        M(t)        TC(t)
                N(t)        TR(t)"));
    iv=seq(from=1,to=nout,by=2);
    for(it in iv){
      cat(sprintf("%10.2f %10.3f %10.3f %10.3f %10.3f\n",
                  tout[it],M[it],TC[it],N[it],TR[it]));
    }
```

- The number of calls to ode1a is displayed at the end of the solution.

```
#
# Calls to ODE routine
  cat(sprintf("\n\n ncall = %5d\n\n",ncall));
```

- The four dependent variable are plotted against t with the R utility plot. The argument type="l" specfied a continuous line (rather than discrete points).

```
#
# Plot ODE solutions
#
# M(t)
  plot(tout,M,xlab="time (days)",ylab="M(t)",
    xlim=c(t0,tf),main="",type="l",lwd=2,
    col="black");
#
# TC(t)
  plot(tout,TC,xlab="time (days)",ylab="TC(t)",
    xlim=c(t0,tf),main="",type="l",lwd=2,
    col="black");
#
# N(t)
  plot(tout,N,xlab="time (days)",ylab="N(t)",
    xlim=c(t0,tf),main="",type="l",lwd=2,
    col="black");
#
# TR(t)
  plot(tout,TR,xlab="time (days)",ylab="TR(t)",
    xlim=c(t0,tf),main="",type="l",lwd=2,
    col="black");
```

This completes the discussion of the main program of Listing 1.1. The subordinate routine ode1a called by ODE integrator lsodes is considered next.

(1.1.2)   ODE routine

```
         Listing 1.2: ODE routine ode1a for eqs. (1.1), (1.2)
  ode1a=function(t,y,parms){
#
# Function ode1a computes the t derivatives
# of M(t),TC(t),N(t),TR(t)
#
# One vector to four scalars
   M=y[1];
  TC=y[2];
   N=y[3];
  TR=y[4];
#
# ODEs
  Mt=sM+rM*(1-M/KM)*M-
     delM*(1+(aNM*N/(bNM+N)+aCM*TC/(bCM+TC)+
     aCNM*N/(bNM+N)*TC/(bCM+TC))*(1-aMM*M/(bMM+M)-
     aRM*TR/(bRM+TR)))*M;
  TCt=rC*(1-TC/KC)*(1+aMC*M/(bMC+M)+aNC*TR/(bRM+TR))*TC-
     delC*TC;
  Nt=sN+rN*(1-N/KN)*(1+aCN*TC/(bCN+TC))*N-delN*N;
  TRt=rR*(1-TR/KR)*(1+aMR*M/(bMR+M))*TR-delR*TR;
#
# Four scalars to one vector
  yt=rep(0,4);
  yt[1]=Mt;
  yt[2]=TCt;
  yt[3]=Nt;
  yt[4]=TRt;
#
# Increment calls to ode1a
  ncall <<- ncall+1;
#
# Return derivative vector
  return(list(c(yt)));
  }
```

We can note the following details about the ODE programming of Listing 1.2.

- The function is defined.

```
ode1a=function(t,y,parms){
#
# Function ode1a computes the t derivatives
# of M(t),TC(t),N(t),TR(t)
```

  t is the current value of t in eqs. (1.1). y is the 4-vector of ODE dependent variables. parms is an argument to pass parameters to ode1a (unused, but required in the argument list). The arguments must be listed in the order stated to properly interface with lsodes called in the main program of Listing 1.1. The derivative vector of the LHS of eqs. (1.1) is calculated and returned to lsodes as explained subsequently.
- Vector y is placed in four scalars to facilitate the programming of eqs. (1.1).

```
#
# One vector to four scalars
    M=y[1];
   TC=y[2];
    N=y[3];
   TR=y[4];
```

- Equation (1.1-1) is programmed $\left(\text{Mt} = \dfrac{dM}{dt} \right)$.

```
#
# ODEs
    Mt=sM+rM*(1-M/KM)*M-
       delM*(1+(aNM*N/(bNM+N)+aCM*TC/(bCM+TC)+
       aCNM*N/(bNM+N)*TC/(bCM+TC))*(1-aMM*M/(bMM+M)-
       aRM*TR/(bRM+TR)))*M;
```

The parameters (constants) defined in the main program of Listing 1.1 are available to ode1a without any special designation (a feature of R). Also, lines can be continued onto second lines without any special designation (a feature of R), but a character at the end of the first line indicating a continuation is recommended (e.g., the first line ends in – indicating a continuation onto a second line). This is a better procedure than placing the – at the beginning of the second line.

- Equation (1.1-2) is programmed $\left(\text{TCt} = \dfrac{dT_C}{dt} \right)$.

  ```
  TCt=rC*(1-TC/KC)*(1+aMC*M/(bMC+M)+aNC*TR/(bRM+TR))*TC-
    delC*TC;
  ```

- Equation (1.1-3) is programmed $\left(\text{Nt} = \dfrac{dN}{dt} \right)$.

  ```
  Nt=sN+rN*(1-N/KN)*(1+aCN*TC/(bCN+TC))*N-delN*N;
  ```

- Equation (1.1-4) is programmed $\left(\text{TRt} = \dfrac{dT_R}{dt} \right)$.

  ```
  TRt=rR*(1-TR/KR)*(1+aMR*M/(bMR+M))*TR-delR*TR;
  ```

- With the completion of the four LHS t derivatives of eqs. (1.1), the derivatives are placed in a vector yt for return to lsodes.

  ```
  #
  # Four scalars to one vector
    yt=rep(0,4);
    yt[1]=Mt;
    yt[2]=TCt;
    yt[3]=Nt;
    yt[4]=TRt;
  ```

- The counter for the calls to ode1a is incremented and returned to the main program of Listing 1.1 by <<-.

  ```
  #
  # Increment calls to ode1a
    ncall <<- ncall+1;
  ```

- The vector yt is returned to lsodes for the next step along the solution.

  ```
  #
  # Return derivative vector
    return(list(c(yt)));
    }
  ```

  The vector yt is returned as a list as required by lsodes. c is the R vector utility. The final } concludes ode1a.

This completes the discussion of ode1a. The output from the main program of Listing 1.1 and ODE routine ode1a of Listing 1.2 is considered next.

(1.1.3) Numerical, graphical output

The numerical output is in Table 1.4.

We can note the following details about this output.

- 41 t output points as the first dimension of the solution matrix out from lsodes as programmed in the main program of Listing 1.1 (with nout=41).
- The solution matrix out returned by lsodes has 5 elements as a second dimension. The first element is the value of t. Elements 2 to 5 are $M(t), T_C(t), N(t), T_R(t)$ from eqs. (1.1) (for each of the 41 output points).

Table 1.4: Abbreviated output from Listings 1.1, 1.2

[1] 41

[1] 5

t	M(t)	TC(t)	N(t)	TR(t)
0.00	4.000	464.000	227.000	42.000
50.00	4.334	520.253	264.319	46.477
100.00	4.570	533.274	272.048	46.922
150.00	4.747	537.642	273.483	47.210
200.00	4.879	540.026	273.815	47.413
250.00	4.976	541.615	273.940	47.557
300.00	5.047	542.722	274.011	47.659
350.00	5.098	543.499	274.058	47.730
400.00	5.135	544.044	274.091	47.781
450.00	5.160	544.427	274.114	47.816
500.00	5.179	544.695	274.130	47.841
550.00	5.192	544.883	274.141	47.859
600.00	5.201	545.015	274.149	47.871
650.00	5.207	545.107	274.155	47.879
700.00	5.211	545.172	274.159	47.885
750.00	5.215	545.217	274.161	47.890
800.00	5.217	545.248	274.163	47.892
850.00	5.218	545.270	274.165	47.895
900.00	5.219	545.286	274.165	47.896
950.00	5.220	545.297	274.166	47.897
1000.00	5.221	545.304	274.167	47.898

ncall =   131

- The solution is displayed for $t = 0, 50, ..., 1000$ as programmed in Listing 1.1 (every second value of t displayed as explained previously).
- ICs (1.2) are confirmed ($t = 0$).
- $M(t), T_C(t), N(t), T_R(t)$ approach an equilibrium (steady state) solution as $t \rightarrow 1000$.
- The computational effort as indicated by `ncall = 131` is modest so that `lsodes` computed the solution to eqs. (1.1) efficiently.

The graphical output is in Figures 1.1.

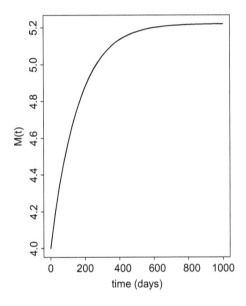

Figure 1.1-1: Numerical solution $M(t)$ from eq. (1.1-1).

Figures 1.1 confirm the solutions in Table 1.4. In particular, the ICs (1.2) and the approach to an equilibrium solution are clear.

(1.2)   Summary and conclusions

The R programming for eqs. (1.1), (1.2) is straightforward through the use of the library initial value ODE integrator `lsodes`. The approach to the equilibrium solution could be confirmed further by displaying the t derivatives (from `ode1a`), $\frac{dM(t)}{dt}, \frac{dT_C(t)}{dt}, \frac{dN(t)}{dt}, \frac{dT_R(t)}{dt}$ which approach zero for large t. This is left as an exercise.

Equations (1.1) are derived as mass balances on the peripheral blood [2]. The model is now extended in Chapter 2 to the bone marrow represented in

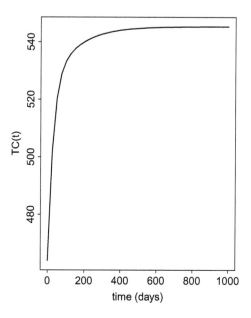

Figure 1.1-2: Numerical solution $T_C(t)$ from eq. (1.1-2).

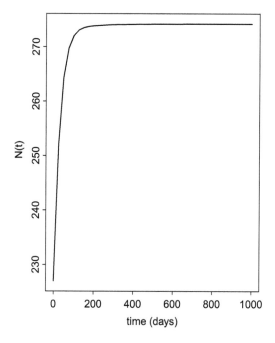

Figure 1.1-3: Numerical solution $N(t)$ from eq. (1.1-3).

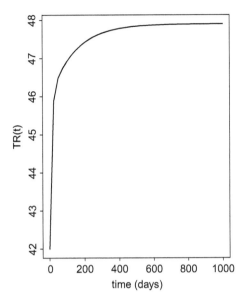

Figure 1.1-4: Numerical solution $T_R(t)$ from eq. (1.1-4).

1D cylindrical coordinates. The radial coordinate r is added to t as an independent variable so that partial differential equations (PDEs) are the basic mathematical form of the model, with dependent variables $M(r,t)$, $T_C(r,t)$, $N(r,t)$, $T_R(r,t)$.

References

1. American Chemical Society, `https://www.cancer.org/cancer/multiple-myeloma/about/what-is-multiple-myeloma.html`.
2. Gallaher, J., et al. (2018), A Mathematical Model for TumorImmune Dynamics in Multiple Myeloma, *Understanding Complex Biological Systems with Mathematics*, A. Radunskaya, R. Segal, and B. Shtylla (eds.), Association for Women in Mathematics Series, vol. 14, Chapter 5, pp. 89–122, Springer, Cham.
3. Gallaher, J., et al. (2018), Methods for determining key components in a mathematical model for tumor-immune dynamics in multiple myeloma, *Journal of Theoretical Biology*, **458**, pp. 31–46.
4. Soetaert, K., J. Cash, and F. Mazzia (2012), *Solving Differential Equations in R*, Springer-Verlag, Heidelberg, Germany.

2 Basic PDE Model

(2) Introduction

The ODE model discussed in Chapter 1 does not take into account spatial distribution of the four dependent variables, $M(t), T_C(t), N(t), T_R(t)$. To accomplish this, one or more spatial independent variables (coordinates) must be included. In the subsequent analysis, the bone marrow, which is the source of the four dependent variable components (Table 1.1), is approximated spatially as a 1D cylinder with the radial coordinate r (in the 3D cylindrical coordinate system (r, θ, z)).

(2.1) PDE model

The following partial differential equations (PDEs) are the ODEs of eqs. (1.1) with a radial diffusion term added to the RHSs.

$$\frac{\partial M}{\partial t} = D_M \left(\frac{\partial^2 M}{\partial r^2} + \frac{1}{r} \frac{\partial M}{\partial r} \right) + s_M + r_M \left(1 - \frac{M}{K_M} \right) M$$

$$- \delta_M \left[1 + \left(\frac{a_{NM} N}{b_{NM} + N} + \frac{a_{CM} T_C}{b_{CM} + T_C} + a_{CNM} \frac{N}{b_{NM} + N} \cdot \frac{T_C}{b_{CM} + T_C} \right) \cdot \right.$$

$$\left. \left(1 - \frac{a_{MM} M}{b_{MM} + M} - \frac{a_{RM} T_R}{b_{RM} + T_R} \right) \right] \cdot M \qquad (2.1\text{-}1)$$

$$\frac{\partial T_C}{\partial t} = D_{T_C} \left(\frac{\partial^2 T_C}{\partial r^2} + \frac{1}{r} \frac{\partial T_C}{\partial r} \right)$$

$$+ r_C \left(1 - \frac{T_C}{K_C} \right) \left(1 + \frac{a_{MC} M}{b_{MC} + M} + \frac{a_{NC} N}{b_{NC} + N} \right) T_C - \delta_C T_C \qquad (2.1\text{-}2)$$

$$\frac{\partial N}{\partial t} = D_N \left(\frac{\partial^2 N}{\partial r^2} + \frac{1}{r} \frac{\partial N}{\partial r} \right)$$

$$+ s_N + r_N \left(1 - \frac{N}{K_N} \right) \left(1 + \frac{a_{CN} T_C}{b_{CN} + T_C} \right) N - \delta_N N \qquad (2.1\text{-}3)$$

$$\frac{\partial T_R}{\partial t} = D_{T_R} \left(\frac{\partial^2 T_R}{\partial r^2} + \frac{1}{r} \frac{\partial T_R}{\partial r} \right)$$

$$+ r_R \left(1 - \frac{T_R}{K_R} \right) \left(1 + \frac{a_{MR} M}{b_{MR} + M} \right) T_R - \delta_R T_R \qquad (2.1\text{-}4)$$

where r is the radial coordinate in the bone marrow. The numerical solutions of eqs. (2.1) are $M(r,t)$, $T_C(r,t)$, $N(r,t)$, $T_R(r,t)$, that is, functions of r and t.

The diffusivities for the four components $M(r,t)$, $T_C(r,t)$, $N(r,t)$, $T_R(r,t)$ in eqs. (2.1) are $D_M, D_{T_C}, D_N, D_{T_R}$.

Equations (2.1) are first order in t and second order in r so they each require one IC and two BCs.

$$M(r, t = 0) = M^0 = 4 \tag{2.2-1}$$

$$T_C(r, t = 0) = T_C^0 = 464 \tag{2.2-2}$$

$$N(r, t = 0) = N^0 = 227 \tag{2.2-3}$$

$$T_R(r, t = 0) = T_R^0 = 42 \tag{2.2-4}$$

$$\frac{\partial M(r = r_l, t)}{\partial r} = \frac{\partial M(r = r_u, t)}{\partial r} = 0 \tag{2.3-1,2}$$

$$\frac{\partial T_C(r = r_l, t)}{\partial r} = \frac{\partial T_C(r = r_u, t)}{\partial r} = 0 \tag{2.3-3,4}$$

$$\frac{\partial N(r = r_l, t)}{\partial r} = \frac{\partial N(r = r_u, t)}{\partial r} = 0 \tag{2.3-5,6}$$

$$\frac{\partial T_R(r = r_l, t)}{\partial r} = \frac{\partial T_R(r = r_u, t)}{\partial r} = 0 \tag{2.3-7,8}$$

Equations (2.3) are homogeneous Neumann BCs.[1] Equations (2.3-1,3,5,7) specify symmetry at $r = r_l = 0$. Equations (2.3-2,4,6,8) specify a zero flux at the outer bone marrow boundary, $r = r_u$. In Chapter 3, BCs (2.3-2,4,6,8) are replaced with Robin BCs that equate the fluxes at the outer boundary to the mass transfer rates between the bone marrow and the peripheral blood. For the following analysis, the zero flux conditions are used to test the programming of the PDE model of eqs. (2.1). In particular, the diffusion terms at $r = r_l = 0$, for example, $\frac{1}{r}\frac{\partial M}{\partial r}$ in eq. (2.1-1), are indeterminate (0/0) and require regularization via l'Hospital's rule. These computational details are explained as the following R routines are discussed, starting with a main program.

---

[1] A Neumann BC specifies the first spatial derivative of the dependent variable at the boundary. A Dirichlet BC specifies the dependent variable at the boundary. A Robin BC specifies the first derivative of the dependent variable as a function of the dependent variable.

(2.1.1) Main program

A main program for eqs. (2.1) through (2.3) follows in Listing 2.1.

Listing 2.1: Main program for eqs. (2.1) through (2.3)

```
#
#  Four PDE MM model
#
# Delete previous workspaces
  rm(list=ls(all=TRUE))
#
# Access ODE integrator
  library("deSolve");
#
# Access functions for numerical solution
  setwd("f:/multipleMyeloma/chap2");
  source("pde1a.R");
  source("dss004.R");
  source("dss044.R");
#
# Select case
#
# ncase-1: Uniform ICs
#
# ncase=2: Gaussian ICs
#
  ncase=2;
#
# Parameters
#
# Eq. (1.1-1)
  sM = 0.001; rM = 0.0175; KM = 10;
  delM = 0.002; aNM = 5; bNM = 150;
  aCM = 5; bCM = 375; aCNM = 8;
  aMM = 0.5; bMM = 3; aRM = 0.5;
  bRM = 25;
#
# Eq. (1.1-2)
  rC =0.013; KC = 800; aMC = 5;
  bMC = 3; aNC = 1; bNC = 150;
  delC = 0.02;
```

(Continued)

Listing 2.1 (Continued): Main program for eqs. (2.1) through (2.3)

```
#
# Eq. (1.1-3)
  sN = 0.03; rN = 0.04; KN = 450;
  aCN = 1; bCN= 375; delN = 0.025;
#
# Eq. (1.1-4)
  rR = 0.0831; KR = 80; aMR = 2;
  bMR = 3; delR = 0.0757;
#
# Diffusivities (cm^2/days)
  days=60*60*24;
   DM=1.0e-09*days;
  DTC=1.0e-09*days;
   DN=1.0e-09*days;
  DTR=1.0e-09*days;
#
# Spatial grid
  rl=0; ru=1; nr=21; dr=(ru-rl)/(nr-1);
  r=seq(from=rl,to=ru,by=dr);
#
# Independent variable for ODE integration
  t0=0;tf=1.0e+03;nout=41;dt=(tf-t0)/(nout-1);
  tout=seq(from=t0,to=tf,by=dt);
#
# Initial conditions (t=0)
  u0=rep(0,4*nr);
  for(ir in 1:nr){
    if(ncase==1){
      u0[ir]       =4;
      u0[ir+nr]   =464;
      u0[ir+2*nr]=227;
      u0[ir+3*nr]= 42;
    }
    if(ncase==2){
      u0[ir]       =4*exp(-25*r[ir]^2);
      u0[ir+nr]   =464*exp(-25*r[ir]^2);
      u0[ir+2*nr]=227*exp(-25*r[ir]^2);
      u0[ir+3*nr]= 42*exp(-25*r[ir]^2);
    }
  }
```

(Continued)

Listing 2.1 (Continued): Main program for eqs. (2.1) through (2.3)

```
  ncall=0;
#
# PDE integration
  out=lsodes(y=u0,times=tout,func=pde1a,
      sparsetype ="sparseint",rtol=1e-6,
      atol=1e-6,maxord=5);
  nrow(out)
  ncol(out)
#
# Arrays for plotting numerical solution
   M=matrix(0,nrow=nr,ncol=nout);
  TC=matrix(0,nrow=nr,ncol=nout);
   N=matrix(0,nrow=nr,ncol=nout);
  TR=matrix(0,nrow=nr,ncol=nout);
  for(it in 1:nout){
  for(ir in 1:nr){
     M[ir,it]=out[it,ir+1];
    TC[ir,it]=out[it,ir+nr+1];
     N[ir,it]=out[it,ir+2*nr+1];
    TR[ir,it]=out[it,ir+3*nr+1];
  }
  }
#
# Display numerical solution
  iv=seq(from=1,to=nout,by=4);
  for(it in iv){
  cat(sprintf("\n\n      t         r         M(t)       TC(t)
                N(t)        TR(t)"));
  iv=seq(from=1,to=nr,by=5);
  for(ir in iv){
    cat(sprintf("\n%6.2f %6.2f %10.3f %10.3f %10.3f %10.3f",
      tout[it],r[ir],M[ir,it],TC[ir,it],N[ir,it],TR[ir,it]));
  }
  }
#
# Calls to ODE routine
  cat(sprintf("\n\n ncall = %5d\n\n",ncall));
```

(Continued)

Listing 2.1 (Continued): Main program for eqs. (2.1) through (2.3)

```
#
# Plot PDE solutions
  par(mfrow=c(1,1));
#
# M(r,t)
#
# 2D
  matplot(r,M,type="l",xlab="r",ylab="M(r,t)",
          lty=1,main="",lwd=2,col="black");
#
# 3D
  persp(r,tout,M,theta=30,phi=30,
        xlim=c(rl,ru),ylim=c(t0,tf),xlab="r",
        ylab="t",zlab="M(r,t)");
#
# TC(r,t)
#
# 2D
  matplot(r,TC,type="l",xlab="r",ylab="TC(r,t)",
          lty=1,main="",lwd=2,col="black");
#
# 3D
  persp(r,tout,TC,theta=30,phi=30,
        xlim=c(rl,ru),ylim=c(t0,tf),xlab="r",
        ylab="t",zlab="TC(r,t)");
#
# N(r,t)
#
# 2D
  matplot(r,N,type="l",xlab="r",ylab="N(r,t)",
          lty=1,main="",lwd=2,col="black");
#
# 3D
  persp(r,tout,N,theta=30,phi=30,
        xlim=c(rl,ru),ylim=c(t0,tf),xlab="r",
        ylab="t",zlab="N(r,t)");
```

(Continued)

**Listing 2.1 (Continued): Main program for eqs. (2.1)
through (2.3)**

```
#
# TR(r,t)
#
# 2D
  matplot(r,TR,type="l",xlab="r",ylab="TR(r,t)",
          lty=1,main="",lwd=2,col="black");
#
# 3D
  persp(r,tout,TR,theta=30,phi=30,
        xlim=c(rl,ru),ylim=c(t0,tf),xlab="r",
        ylab="t",zlab="TR(r,t)");
```

The following discussion of Listing 2.1 parallels the discussion of Listing 1.1
with some repetition that is included so the discussion of the PDE routines is
self-contained.

- Previous workspaces are deleted.

```
#
#  Four PDE MM model
#
# Delete previous workspaces
  rm(list=ls(all=TRUE))
```

- The R ODE integrator library deSolve is accessed. Then the directory with the files for the solution of eqs. (2.1) through (2.3) is
  designated. Note that setwd (set working directory) uses / rather
  than the usual \.

```
#
# Access ODE integrator
  library("deSolve");
#
# Access functions for numerical solution
  setwd("f:/multipleMyeloma/chap2");
  source("pde1a.R");
  source("dss004.R");
  source("dss044.R");
```

pde1a.R is the routine for eqs. (2.1), (2.3) based on the method of lines (MOL), a general algorithm for partial differential equations [4] (discussed subsequently). dss004, dss044 are library routines for the calculation of first and second spatial derivatives. These routines are listed in Appendix A1 with additional explanation.

- ncase selects the IC functions in eqs. (2.2).

```
#
# Select case
#
# ncase-1: Uniform ICs
#
# ncase=2: Gaussian ICs
#
  ncase=2;
```

- The model parameters are specified numerically.

```
#
# Parameters
#
# Eq. (1.1-1)
  sM = 0.001; rM = 0.0175; KM = 10;
  delM = 0.002; aNM = 5; bNM = 150;
  aCM = 5; bCM = 375; aCNM = 8;
  aMM = 0.5; bMM = 3; aRM = 0.5;
  bRM = 25;
#
# Eq. (1.1-2)
  rC =0.013; KC = 800; aMC = 5;
  bMC = 3; aNC = 1; bNC = 150;
  delC = 0.02;
#
# Eq. (1.1-3)
  sN = 0.03; rN = 0.04; KN = 450;
  aCN = 1; bCN= 375; delN = 0.025;
#
# Eq. (1.1-4)
  rR = 0.0831; KR = 80; aMR = 2;
  bMR = 3; delR = 0.0757;
```

- The diffusivities in eqs. (2.1) are defined numerically.

```
#
# Diffusivities (cm^2/days)
```

```
days=60*60*24;
 DM=1.0e-09*days;
DTC=1.0e-09*days;
 DN=1.0e-09*days;
DTR=1.0e-09*days;
```

These diffusivities are based on a representative value for a large molecule in a diffusion restricted medium, `1.0e-09` cm^2/sec, converted to t units of days.
- A spatial grid is defined for r.

```
#
# Spatial grid
  rl=0; ru=1; nr=21; dr=(ru-rl)/(nr-1);
  r=seq(from=rl,to=ru,by=dr);
```

The grid values are $r = 0, 0.05, ..., 1$ cm.
- An interval in t of 41 points is defined for $0 \le t \le 1000$ so that `tout=0,1000/40,...,1000`.

```
#
# Independent variable for ODE integration
  t0=0;tf=1.0e+03;nout=41;dt=(tf-t0)/(nout-1);
  tout=seq(from=t0,to=tf,by=dt);
```

- ICs (1.2) are defined (from [1,2]).

```
#
# Initial conditions (t=0)
  u0=rep(0,4*nr);
  for(ir in 1:nr){
    if(ncase==1){
      u0[ir]       =4;
      u0[ir+nr]   =464;
      u0[ir+2*nr]=227;
      u0[ir+3*nr]= 42;
    }
    if(ncase==2){
      u0[ir]       =4*exp(-25*r[ir]^2);
      u0[ir+nr]   =464*exp(-25*r[ir]^2);
      u0[ir+2*nr]=227*exp(-25*r[ir]^2);
      u0[ir+3*nr]= 42*exp(-25*r[ir]^2);
    }
  }
  ncall=0;
```

For `ncase=1`, the ICs of eqs. (2.2) are constant in r. For `ncase=2` the ICs are Gaussian functions center at $r = r_l = 0$. Also, the counter for the calls to `ode1a` is initialized.

- The system of $4 \times 21 = 84$ ODEs is integrated by the library integrator `lsodes` (available in `deSolve`, [4]). As expected, the inputs to `lsodes` are the ODE function, `pde1a`, the IC vector `u0`, and the vector of output values of t, `tout`. The length of `u0` (84) informs `lsodes` how many ODEs are to be integrated. `func,y,times` are reserved names.

```
#
# PDE integration
  out=lsodes(y=u0,times=tout,func=pde1a,
      sparsetype ="sparseint",rtol=1e-6,
      atol=1e-6,maxord=5);
  nrow(out)
  ncol(out)
```

The designation of sparse matrix integration, `sparsetype = "sparseint"`, is particularly important since the ODE Jacobian matrix of size $84 \times 84 = 7056$ is relatively large and only the nonzero elements are used in the numerical integration with the sparse matrix option. Each of the 84 ODEs is integrated with relative and absolute errors specified with `rtol=1e-6,atol=1e-6` (these are the default values for `lsodes`, but are included here to emphasize the numerical integration error tolerances).

Also, the numerical integration in `lsodes` adjusts the order of the integration algorithm, starting with first order (the implicit Euler method) and possibly reaching fifth order (the default maximum order is 5 and is also specified with `maxord=5`).

- The numerical $M(r,t)$, $T_C(r,t)$, $N(r,t)$, $T_R(r,t)$ from `lsodes` are placed in matrices `M,TC,N,TR` for numerical and graphical display.

```
#
# Arrays for plotting numerical solution
   M=matrix(0,nrow=nr,ncol=nout);
  TC=matrix(0,nrow=nr,ncol=nout);
   N=matrix(0,nrow=nr,ncol=nout);
  TR=matrix(0,nrow=nr,ncol=nout);
  for(it in 1:nout){
  for(ir in 1:nr){
     M[ir,it]=out[it,ir+1];
```

```
      TC[ir,it]=out[it,ir+nr+1];
       N[ir,it]=out[it,ir+2*nr+1];
      TR[ir,it]=out[it,ir+3*nr+1];
    }
    }
```

The offset +1 is required since t is the first element in each solution vector in matrix out. The 2 to 85 elements are the solutions to the 84 ODEs that approximate the four PDEs, eqs. (2.1), by the MOL algorithm (discussed subsequently).

- Abbreviated numerical solutions of eqs. (2.1) are displayed (for every fourth value of t and every fifth value of r with by=4,5).

```
#
# Display numerical solution
  iv=seq(from=1,to=nout,by=4);
  for(it in iv){
  cat(sprintf("\n\n      t      r         M(t)        TC(t)
                N(t)       TR(t)"));
  iv=seq(from=1,to=nr,by=5);
  for(ir in iv){
    cat(sprintf("\n%6.2f %6.2f %10.3f %10.3f %10.3f %10.3f",
    tout[it],r[ir],M[ir,it],TC[ir,it],N[ir,it],TR[ir,it]));
  }
  }
```

- The counter for the calls to pde1a is displayed at the end of the solution.

```
#
# Calls to ODE routine
  cat(sprintf("\n\n ncall = %5d\n\n",ncall));
```

- $M(r,t)$, $T_C(r,t)$, $N(r,t)$, $T_R(r,t)$ are plotted in 2D with matplot and in 3D with persp.

```
#
# Plot PDE solutions
  par(mfrow=c(1,1));
#
# M(r,t)
#
```

```
# 2D
  matplot(r,M,type="l",xlab="r",ylab="M(r,t)",
          lty=1,main="",lwd=2,col="black");
#
# 3D
  persp(r,tout,M,theta=30,phi=30,
        xlim=c(rl,ru),ylim=c(t0,tf),xlab="r",
        ylab="t",zlab="M(r,t)");
#
# TC(r,t)
#
# 2D
  matplot(r,TC,type="l",xlab="r",ylab="TC(r,t)",
          lty=1,main="",lwd=2,col="black");
#
# 3D
  persp(r,tout,TC,theta=30,phi=30,
        xlim=c(rl,ru),ylim=c(t0,tf),xlab="r",
        ylab="t",zlab="TC(r,t)");
#
# N(r,t)
#
# 2D
  matplot(r,N,type="l",xlab="r",ylab="N(r,t)",
          lty=1,main="",lwd=2,col="black");
#
# 3D
  persp(r,tout,N,theta=30,phi=30,
        xlim=c(rl,ru),ylim=c(t0,tf),xlab="r",
        ylab="t",zlab="N(r,t)");
#
# TR(r,t)
#
# 2D
  matplot(r,TR,type="l",xlab="r",ylab="TR(r,t)",
          lty=1,main="",lwd=2,col="black");
#
# 3D
  persp(r,tout,TR,theta=30,phi=30,
        xlim=c(rl,ru),ylim=c(t0,tf),xlab="r",
        ylab="t",zlab="TR(r,t)");
```

This completes the discussion of the main program of Listing 2.1. The ODE/MOL routine pde1a follows.

(2.1.2) ODE/MOL routine

The ODE/MOL routine for eqs. (1.2) follows in Listing 2.2.

**Listing 2.2: ODE/MOL routine pde1a for eqs. (2.1)
through (2.3)**

```
  pde1a=function(t,u,parm){
#
# Function pde1a computes the t derivative
# vector of M(r,t), TR(r,t), N(r,t), TR(r,t)
#
# One vector to four vectors
   M=rep(0,nr);
  TC=rep(0,nr);
   N=rep(0,nr);
  TR=rep(0,nr);
  for(ir in 1:nr){
     M[ir]=u[ir];
    TC[ir]=u[ir+nr];
     N[ir]=u[ir+2*nr];
    TR[ir]=u[ir+3*nr];
  }
#
# Mr,TCr,Nr,TRr
   Mr=dss004(rl,ru,nr, M);
  TCr=dss004(rl,ru,nr,TC);
   Nr=dss004(rl,ru,nr, N);
  TRr=dss004(rl,ru,nr,TR);
#
# BCs
   Mr[1]=0;   Mr[nr]=0;
  TCr[1]=0;  TCr[nr]=0;
   Nr[1]=0;   Nr[nr]=0;
  TRr[1]=0;  TRr[nr]=0;
#
# Mrr,TCrr,Nrr,TRrr
  nl=2;nu=2;
   Mrr=dss044(rl,ru,nr, M, Mr,nl,nu);
  TCrr=dss044(rl,ru,nr,TC,TCr,nl,nu);
   Nrr=dss044(rl,ru,nr, N, Nr,nl,nu);
  TRrr=dss044(rl,ru,nr,TR,TRr,nl,nu);
#
# PDEs
   Mt=rep(0,nr);
```

(Continued)

Listing 2.2 (Continued): ODE/MOL routine pde1a for eqs. (2.1) through (2.3)

```
TCt=rep(0,nr);
 Nt=rep(0,nr);
TRt=rep(0,nr);
for(ir in 1:nr){
  if(ir==1){
    Mt[ir]=DM*2*Mrr[ir]+
           sM+rM*(1-M[ir]/KM)*M[ir]-
           delM*(1+(aNM*N[ir]/(bNM+N[ir])+
           aCM*TC[ir]/(bCM+TC[ir])+
           aCNM*N[ir]/(bNM+N[ir])*TC[ir]/(bCM+TC[ir]))*
           (1-aMM*M[ir]/(bMM+M[ir])-
           aRM*TR[ir]/(bRM+TR[ir])))*M[ir];
    TCt[ir]=DTC*2*TCrr[ir]+
           rC*(1-TC[ir]/KC)*(1+aMC*M[ir]/(bMC+M[ir])+
           aNC*TR[ir]/(bRM+TR[ir]))*TC[ir]-delC*TC[ir];
     Nt[ir]=DN*2*Nrr[ir]+
           sN+rN*(1-N[ir]/KN)*(1+aCN*TC[ir]/(bCN+TC[ir]))*
           N[ir]-delN*N[ir];
    TRt[ir]=DTR*2*TRrr[ir]+
           rR*(1-TR[ir]/KR)*(1+aMR*M[ir]/(bMR+M[ir]))*
           TR[ir]-delR*TR[ir];
  }
  if(ir>1){
    Mt[ir]=DM*(Mrr[ir]+(1/r[ir])*Mr[ir])+
           sM+rM*(1-M[ir]/KM)*M[ir]-
           delM*(1+(aNM*N[ir]/(bNM+N[ir])+
           aCM*TC[ir]/(bCM+TC[ir])+
           aCNM*N[ir]/(bNM+N[ir])*TC[ir]/(bCM+TC[ir]))*
           (1-aMM*M[ir]/(bMM+M[ir])-
           aRM*TR[ir]/(bRM+TR[ir])))*M[ir];
    TCt[ir]=DTC*(TCrr[ir]+(1/r[ir])*TCr[ir])+
           rC*(1-TC[ir]/KC)*(1+aMC*M[ir]/(bMC+M[ir])+
           aNC*TR[ir]/(bRM+TR[ir]))*TC[ir]-delC*TC[ir];
     Nt[ir]=DN*(Nrr[ir]+(1/r[ir])*Nr[ir])+
           sN+rN*(1-N[ir]/KN)*(1+aCN*TC[ir]/(bCN+TC[ir]))*
           N[ir]-delN*N[ir];
    TRt[ir]=DTR*(TRrr[ir]+(1/r[ir])*TRr[ir])+
           rR*(1-TR[ir]/KR)*(1+aMR*M[ir]/(bMR+M[ir]))*
           TR[ir]-delR*TR[ir];
  }
}
```

(Continued)

Listing 2.2 (Continued): ODE/MOL routine pde1a for eqs. (2.1)
through (2.3)

```
#
# Four vectors to one vector
  ut=rep(0,4*nr);
  for(ir in 1:nr){
    ut[ir]     = Mt[ir];
    ut[ir+nr]  =TCt[ir];
    ut[ir+2*nr]= Nt[ir];
    ut[ir+3*nr]=TRt[ir];
  }
#
# Increment calls to pde1a
  ncall<<-ncall+1;
#
# Return derivative vector
  return(list(c(ut)));
}
```

We can note the following details about pde1a.

- The function is defined.

  ```
  pde1a=function(t,u,parm){
  #
  # Function pde1a computes the t derivative
  # vector of M(r,t), TR(r,t), N(r,t), TR(r,t)
  ```

  t is the current value of t in eqs. (2.1). u is the current numerical
  solution to eqs. (2.1) (placed in u in the order of the IC vector,
  u0). parm is an argument to pass parameters to pde1a (unused,
  but required in the argument list). The arguments must be listed
  in the order stated to properly interface with lsodes called in the
  main program of Listing 2.1. The ODE/MOL approximations of
  the derivatives $\frac{\partial M(r,t)}{\partial t}$, $\frac{\partial T_C(r,t)}{\partial t}$, $\frac{\partial N(r,t)}{\partial t}$, $\frac{\partial T_R(r,t)}{\partial t}$ of eqs. (2.1) are
  calculated and returned to lsodes as explained subsequently.

- The dependent variable vector, u, is placed in four vectors to facilitate the programming of eqs. (2.1).

  ```
  #
  # One vector to four vectors
    M=rep(0,nr);
    TC=rep(0,nr);
  ```

```
   N=rep(0,nr);
   TR=rep(0,nr);
   for(ir in 1:nr){
     M[ir]=u[ir];
     TC[ir]=u[ir+nr];
     N[ir]=u[ir+2*nr];
     TR[ir]=u[ir+3*nr];
   }
```

- The first derivatives in eqs. (2.1) $\frac{\partial M(r,t)}{\partial r}$, $\frac{\partial T_C(r,t)}{\partial r}$, $\frac{\partial N(r,t)}{\partial r}$, $\frac{\partial T_R(r,t)}{\partial r}$ are computed with dss004. The arguments of dss004 are explained in Appendix A1.

```
#
# Mr,TCr,Nr,TRr
   Mr=dss004(rl,ru,nr, M);
   TCr=dss004(rl,ru,nr,TC);
   Nr=dss004(rl,ru,nr, N);
   TRr=dss004(rl,ru,nr,TR);
```

- The homogeneous Neumann BCs (2.3) are programmed.

```
#
# BCs
   Mr[1]=0;   Mr[nr]=0;
  TCr[1]=0;  TCr[nr]=0;
   Nr[1]=0;   Nr[nr]=0;
  TRr[1]=0;  TRr[nr]=0;
```

The subscripts 1,nr refer to $r = r_l = 0, r = r_u = 1$, respectively.

- The second derivatives in eqs. (2.1) $\frac{\partial^2 M(r,t)}{\partial r^2}$, $\frac{\partial^2 T_C(r,t)}{\partial r^2}$, $\frac{\partial^2 N(r,t)}{\partial r^2}$, $\frac{\partial^2 T_R(r,t)}{\partial r^2}$ are computed with dss044. The arguments of dss044 are explained in Appendix A1. nl=2,nu=2 specify Neumann BCs at $r = r_l = 0, r = r_u = 1$, respectively.

```
#
# Mrr,TCrr,Nrr,TRrr
   nl=2;nu=2;
    Mrr=dss044(rl,ru,nr, M, Mr,nl,nu);
   TCrr=dss044(rl,ru,nr,TC,TCr,nl,nu);
    Nrr=dss044(rl,ru,nr, N, Nr,nl,nu);
   TRrr=dss044(rl,ru,nr,TR,TRr,nl,nu);
```

- Equations (2.1) are programmed at $r = 0$ for which the radial group $\frac{1}{r}\frac{\partial}{\partial r}$ is indeterminate (0/0). With the use of BCs (2.3-1,3,5,7) and l'Hospital's rule

$$\frac{1}{r}\frac{\partial}{\partial r}\big|_{r\to 0} = \frac{\partial^2}{\partial r^2}$$

so that, for example, the radial group in eq. (2.1-1) is

$$\frac{\partial^2 M}{\partial r^2} + \frac{1}{r}\frac{\partial M}{\partial r}\big|_{r\to 0} = 2\frac{\partial^2 M}{\partial r^2}$$

which is programmed as 2*Mrr[ir]. Note that the four dependent variables (Table 1.1) are now vectors with subscript [ir] which indicates the approximation of PDEs (2.1) with nr ODEs. This is essentially the MOL.

```
#
# PDEs
  Mt=rep(0,nr);
  TCt=rep(0,nr);
  Nt=rep(0,nr);
  TRt=rep(0,nr);
  for(ir in 1:nr){
    if(ir==1){
      Mt[ir]=DM*2*Mrr[ir]+
             sM+rM*(1-M[ir]/KM)*M[ir]-
             delM*(1+(aNM*N[ir]/(bNM+N[ir])+
             aCM*TC[ir]/(bCM+TC[ir])+
             aCNM*N[ir]/(bNM+N[ir])*TC[ir]/(bCM+TC[ir]))*
             (1-aMM*M[ir]/(bMM+M[ir])-
             aRM*TR[ir]/(bRM+TR[ir])))*M[ir];
      TCt[ir]=DTC*2*TCrr[ir]+
             rC*(1-TC[ir]/KC)*(1+aMC*M[ir]/(bMC+M[ir])+
             aNC*TR[ir]/(bRM+TR[ir]))*TC[ir]-delC*TC[ir];
      Nt[ir]=DN*2*Nrr[ir]+
             sN+rN*(1-N[ir]/KN)*(1+aCN*TC[ir]/(bCN+
             TC[ir]))*N[ir]-delN*N[ir];
      TRt[ir]=DTR*2*TRrr[ir]+
             rR*(1-TR[ir]/KR)*(1+aMR*M[ir]/(bMR+M[ir]))*
             TR[ir]-delR*TR[ir];
    }
```

- For $r > 0$, eqs. (2.1) are programmed directly in the MOL format.

```
    if(ir>1){
      Mt[ir]=DM*(Mrr[ir]+(1/r[ir])*Mr[ir])+
             sM+rM*(1-M[ir]/KM)*M[ir]-
```

```
         delM*(1+(aNM*N[ir]/(bNM+N[ir])+
         aCM*TC[ir]/(bCM+TC[ir])+
         aCNM*N[ir]/(bNM+N[ir])*TC[ir]/(bCM+TC[ir]))*
         (1-aMM*M[ir]/(bMM+M[ir])-
         aRM*TR[ir]/(bRM+TR[ir])))*M[ir];
    TCt[ir]=DTC*(TCrr[ir]+(1/r[ir])*TCr[ir])+
         rC*(1-TC[ir]/KC)*(1+aMC*M[ir]/(bMC+M[ir])+
         aNC*TR[ir]/(bRM+TR[ir]))*TC[ir]-delC*TC[ir];
     Nt[ir]=DN*(Nrr[ir]+(1/r[ir])*Nr[ir])+
         sN+rN*(1-N[ir]/KN)*(1+aCN*TC[ir]/(bCN+
         TC[ir]))*N[ir]-delN*N[ir];
    TRt[ir]=DTR*(TRrr[ir]+(1/r[ir])*TRr[ir])+
         rR*(1-TR[ir]/KR)*(1+aMR*M[ir]/(bMR+M[ir]))*
         TR[ir]-delR*TR[ir];
   }
 }
```

The final } concludes pde1a.

- The four t derivative vectors (LHS of eqs. (2.1)) are placed in a single vector ut to return to lsodes for the next step along the solution.

```
#
# Four vectors to one vector
  ut=rep(0,4*nr);
  for(ir in 1:nr){
    ut[ir]      = Mt[ir];
    ut[ir+nr]   =TCt[ir];
    ut[ir+2*nr]= Nt[ir];
    ut[ir+3*nr]=TRt[ir];
  }
```

- The counter for the calls to pde1a is incremented and returned to the main program of Listing 2.1 with <<-.

```
#
# Increment calls to pde1a
  ncall<<-ncall+1;
```

- The t derivative vector ut is returned to lsodes as a list.

```
#
# Return derivative vector
  return(list(c(ut)));
```

c is the R vector operator.

This concludes the discussion of the ODE/MOL routine pde1a. The output from the main program and subordinate routine pde1a of Listings 2.1, 2.2, is considered next.

(2.1.3) Numerical, graphical output

Table 2.1: Abbreviated output for ncase=1

[1] 41

[1] 85

t	r	M(t)	TC(t)	N(t)	TR(t)
0.00	0.00	4.000	464.000	227.000	42.000
0.00	0.25	4.000	464.000	227.000	42.000
0.00	0.50	4.000	464.000	227.000	42.000
0.00	0.75	4.000	464.000	227.000	42.000
0.00	1.00	4.000	464.000	227.000	42.000

t	r	M(t)	TC(t)	N(t)	TR(t)
100.00	0.00	4.570	533.274	272.048	46.922
100.00	0.25	4.570	533.274	272.048	46.922
100.00	0.50	4.570	533.274	272.048	46.922
100.00	0.75	4.570	533.274	272.048	46.922
100.00	1.00	4.570	533.274	272.048	46.922

.

.

.

Output for t = 200,...,900 removed

.

.

.

t	r	M(t)	TC(t)	N(t)	TR(t)
1000.00	0.00	5.221	545.304	274.167	47.898
1000.00	0.25	5.221	545.304	274.167	47.898
1000.00	0.50	5.221	545.304	274.167	47.898
1000.00	0.75	5.221	545.304	274.167	47.898
1000.00	1.00	5.221	545.304	274.167	47.898

ncall =   235

We can note the following details about this output.

- 41 output points in t (from `nout=41` in the main program of Listing 2.1) as the first dimension of the solution matrix `out` from `lsodes`.
- The solution matrix `out` returned by `lsodes` has 85 elements as a second dimension. The first element is the value of t. Elements 2 to 85 in `out` are $M(r,t)$, $T_C(r,t)$, $N(r,t)$, $T_R(r,t)$ for eqs. (2.1).
- The solution is displayed for $t = 0, 100, ..., 1000$ and $r = 0, 0.05, ..., 1$ as programmed in Listing 2.1 (every fourth value of t and every fifth value of r, as discussed previously).
- ICs (2.2) ($t = 0$) are confirmed. This check is important since if the ICs are not correct, the subsequent solution will also not be correct. Note in particular the constant values in r (from the ICs with `ncase=1`).
- The solutions remain invariant (constant) in r which is expected from the homogeneous Neumann BCs (2.3). This may seem like a trivial case, but it is worth considering since a variation of the solutions in r would indicate a programming error.
- The PDE solutions agree with the ODE solutions of Chapter 1, Table 1.4. For example at $t = 1000$

Table 1.4

t	M(t)	TC(t)	N(t)	TR(t)
1000.00	5.221	545.304	274.167	47.898

Table 2.1

t	r	M(t)	TC(t)	N(t)	TR(t)
1000.00	0.00	5.221	545.304	274.167	47.898
1000.00	0.25	5.221	545.304	274.167	47.898
1000.00	0.50	5.221	545.304	274.167	47.898
1000.00	0.75	5.221	545.304	274.167	47.898
1000.00	1.00	5.221	545.304	274.167	47.898

- The computational effort is modest, `ncall = 235`, so that `lsodes` efficiently computed a solution to eqs. (2.1).

The graphical output follows (three figures with `matplot` are not included to conserve space since Figures 2.1-3,5,7 essentially duplicate Figure 2.1-1).

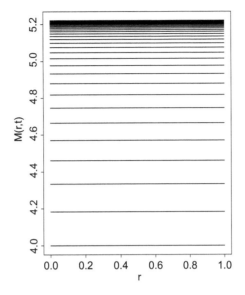

Figure 2.1-1: Numerical solution $M(r,t)$ from eq. (2.1-1), `ncase=1`, `matplot`.

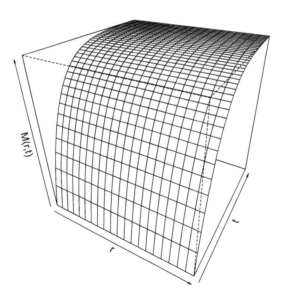

Figure 2.1-2: Numerical solution $M(r,t)$ from eq. (2.1-1), `ncase=1`, `persp`.

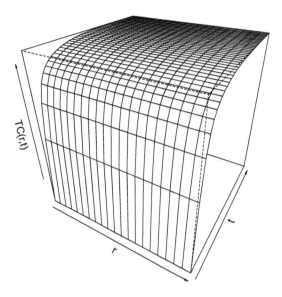

Figure 2.1-4: Numerical solution $T_C(r,t)$ from eq. (2.1-2), `ncase=1`, `persp`.

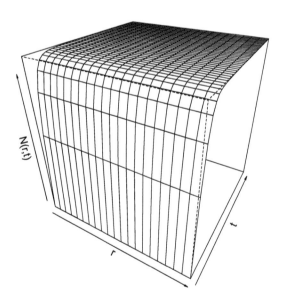

Figure 2.1-6: Numerical solution $N(r,t)$ from eq. (2.1-3), `ncase=1`, `persp`.

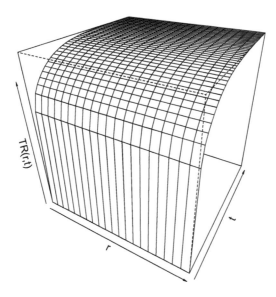

Figure 2.1-8: Numerical solution $T_R(r,t)$ from eq. (2.1-4), ncase=1, persp.

Figures 2.1 generally demonstrate the uniform (constant in r) ICs and approach to an equilibrium (steady state solution).

For ncase=2 (in the main program of Listing 2.1), Gaussian functions are used in ICs (2.2). The output follows.

We can note the following details about this output.

- The Gaussian ICs are confirmed (at $t = 0$).
- The ICs redistribute in r through diffusion, but approach the same equilibrium solutions as for ncase=1 (Table 2.1). In other words, despite the differences in the ICs (constant for ncase=1, Gaussian for ncase=2), the final equilibrium solutions are the same.
- The computational effort remains modest, ncall = 401, so that lsodes efficiently computed a solution to eqs. (2.1).

These features of the solutions are confirmed in Figures 2.2.

Table 2.2: Abbreviated output for ncase=2

```
[1] 41

[1] 85
```

t	r	M(t)	TC(t)	N(t)	TR(t)
0.00	0.00	4.000	464.000	227.000	42.000
0.00	0.25	0.838	97.260	47.582	8.804
0.00	0.50	0.008	0.896	0.438	0.081
0.00	0.75	0.000	0.000	0.000	0.000
0.00	1.00	0.000	0.000	0.000	0.000

t	r	M(t)	TC(t)	N(t)	TR(t)
100.00	0.00	3.195	469.800	254.286	43.768
100.00	0.25	1.903	277.228	182.057	36.203
100.00	0.50	0.477	12.900	26.128	5.791
100.00	0.75	0.238	0.088	7.115	0.048
100.00	1.00	0.233	0.001	6.835	0.000

```
                            .                    .
                            .                    .
                            .                    .
             Output for t = 200,...,900 removed
                            .                    .
                            .                    .
                            .                    .
```

t	r	M(t)	TC(t)	N(t)	TR(t)
1000.00	0.00	5.201	545.026	274.150	47.872
1000.00	0.25	5.202	545.039	274.151	47.873
1000.00	0.50	5.205	545.080	274.153	47.877
1000.00	0.75	5.209	545.136	274.157	47.882
1000.00	1.00	5.211	545.163	274.158	47.885

```
ncall =   401
```

Figures 2.2 demonstrate the diffusion of the four dependent variable components (Table 2.2), including the contribution of the Neumann BCs of eqs. (2.3).

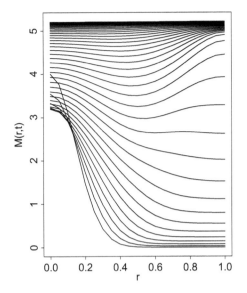

Figure 2.2-1: Numerical solution $M(r, t)$ from eq. (2.1-1), `ncase=2`, `matplot`.

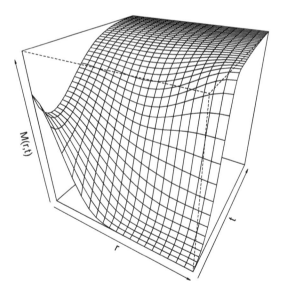

Figure 2.2-2: Numerical solution $M(r, t)$ from eq. (2.1-1), `ncase=2`, `persp`.

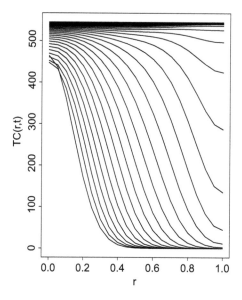

Figure 2.2-3: Numerical solution $T_C(r, t)$ from eq. (2.1-2), `ncase=2`, `matplot`.

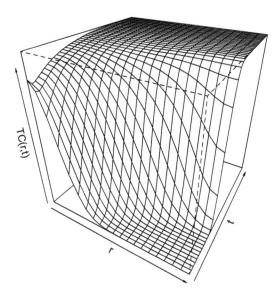

Figure 2.2-4: Numerical solution $T_C(r, t)$ from eq. (2.1-2), `ncase=2`, `persp`.

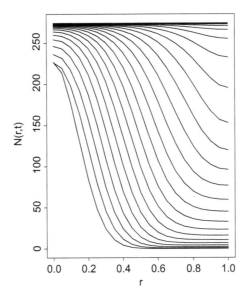

Figure 2.2-5: Numerical solution $N(r, t)$ from eq. (2.1-3), `ncase=2`, `matplot`.

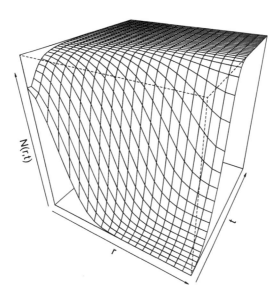

Figure 2.2-6: Numerical solution $N(r, t)$ from eq. (2.1-3), `ncase=2`, `persp`.

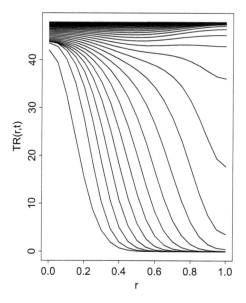

Figure 2.2-7: Numerical solution $T_R(r, t)$ from eq. (2.1-4), `ncase=2`, `matplot`.

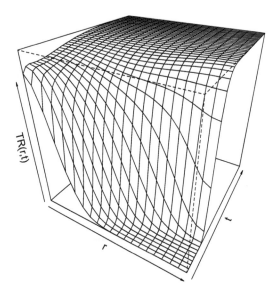

Figure 2.2-8: Numerical solution $T_R(r, t)$ from eq. (2.1-4), `ncase=2`, `persp`.

(2.2) Summary and conclusions

The MOL numerical integration of eqs. (2.1) illustrates (1) the effect of the ICs of eqs. (2.2), including the convergence to the same equilibrium solution that agrees with the solution of the ODE model in Chapter 1, (2) the radial diffusion of the four components (Table 1.1), including the calculation of the radial (spatial) derivatives with homogeneous Neumann BCs of eqs. (2.3), and (3) the programming of the nonlinear interaction (coupling) terms of eqs. (2.1) (Table 1.3).

The PDE model is now extended in Chapter 3 to include transfer of the four dependent variable components from the bone marrow to the peripheral blood (in place of the no flux BCs of eqs. (2.3-2,4,6,8)).

As a word of caution, changes in the model parameters may cause the execution of the R routines in Listings 2.1, 2.2 to generate error messages, or even to fail. Thus, in making changes in the parameters, an incremental approach with small changes is essential. If an execution error or failure occurs, the last change in the parameters may be the cause of the problem.

References

1. Gallaher, J., et al. (2018), A Mathematical Model for TumorImmune Dynamics in Multiple Myeloma, *Understanding Complex Biological Systems with Mathematics*, A. Radunskaya, R. Segal, and B. Shtylla (eds.), Association for Women in Mathematics Series, vol. 14, Chapter 5, pp. 89–122, Springer, Cham.
2. Gallaher, J., et al. (2018), Methods for determining key components in a mathematical model for tumor-immune dynamics in multiple myeloma, *Journal of Theoretical Biology*, **458**, pp. 31–46.
3. Schiesser, W.E. (2016), *Method of Lines PDE Analysis in Biomedical Science and Engineering*, John Wiley & Sons, Hoboken, NJ.
4. Soetaert, K., J. Cash, and F. Mazzia (2012), *Solving Differential Equations in R*, Springer-Verlag, Heidelberg, Germany.

3 PDE Model with External Transfer

(3) Introduction

The PDE model of eqs. (2.1) represents a closed bone marrow system in the sense that the four PDE dependent variable components [1,2] $M(r,t)$, $T_C(r,t)$, $N(r,t)$, $T_R(r,t)$, cannot be transferred to an external region such as the peripheral blood. This property of a closed system results from the homogeneous Neumann (no flux) BCs at the outer boundary, eqs. (2.3-2,4,6,8). To open this system to external transfer of the dependent variable components (Table 1.1), Robin outer boundary conditions replace the no flux BCs.

$$\frac{\partial M(r = r_l, t)}{\partial r} = 0; \quad \frac{\partial M(r = r_u, t)}{\partial r} = k_M (M_p(t) - M(r = r_u, t)) \quad (3.1\text{-}1,2)$$

$$\frac{\partial T_C(r = r_l, t)}{\partial r} = 0; \quad \frac{\partial T_C(r = r_u, t)}{\partial r} = k_{T_C} (T_{Cp}(t) - T_C(r = r_u, t)) \quad (3.1\text{-}3,4)$$

$$\frac{\partial N(r = r_l, t)}{\partial r} = 0; \quad \frac{\partial N(r = r_u, t)}{\partial r} = k_N (N_p(t) - N(r = r_u, t)) \quad (3.1\text{-}5,6)$$

$$\frac{\partial T_R(r = r_l, t)}{\partial r} = 0; \quad \frac{\partial T_R(r = r_u, t)}{\partial r} = k_{T_R} (T_{Rp}(t) - T_R(r = r_u, t)) \quad (3.1\text{-}7,8)$$

where $k_M, k_{T_C}, k_N, k_{T_R}$ are mass transfer coefficients. Equations (3.1-2,4,6,8) are Robin BCs that equate the flux at the outer boundary $r = r_u$ (LHSs) to the transfer rate into an outer region, e.g., the peripheral blood (RHSs).

(3.1) ODE/PDE model

The ODE/PDE model to be analyzed consists of PDEs (2.1), initial conditions (ICs) (2.2) and boundary conditions (3.1) augmented with four ODEs for the peripheral variables $M_p(t), T_{Cp}(t), N_p(t), T_{Rp}(t)$ that track the outer boundary dependent variables $M(r = r_u, t), T_C(r = r_u, t), N(r = r_u, t), T_R(r = r_u, t)$.

$$\frac{dM_p}{dt} = k_M(M_p(t) - M(r = r_u, t)) \tag{3.2-1}$$

$$\frac{dT_{Cp}}{dt} = k_{T_C}(T_{Cp}(t) - T_C(r = r_u, t)) \tag{3.2-2}$$

$$\frac{dN_p}{dt} = k_N(N_p(t) - N(r = r_u, t)) \tag{3.2-3}$$

$$\frac{dT_{Rp}}{dt} = k_{T_R}(T_{Rp}(t) - T_R(r = r_u, t)) \tag{3.2-4}$$

Equation (3.2) are first order in t and require an IC for each equation.

$$M_p(t = 0) = M_p^0 \tag{3.3-1}$$

$$T_{Cp}(t = 0) = T_{Cp}^0 \tag{3.3-2}$$

$$N_p(t = 0) = N_p^0 \tag{3.3-3}$$

$$T_{Rp}(t = 0) = T_{Rp}^0 \tag{3.3-4}$$

where $M_p^0, T_{Cp}^0, N_p^0, T_{Rp}^0$ are specified constants.

Equations (2.1), (2.2), (3.1) through (3.3) constitute an ODE/MOL model that is accommodated within the method of lines (MOL) [3].

(3.1.1) Main program

The main program of Listing 3.1 parallels the main program of Listing 2.1, so only the differences are explained.

- The mass transfer coefficients of eqs. (3.1), (3.2) are added to the parameter specifications (after the diffusivities).

```
#
# Peripheral ODEs
  kM=1; kTC=1;
  kN=1; kTR=1;
```

- Homogeneous ICs are added for eqs. (3.2), (3.3).

```
#
# Initial conditions (t=0)
  u0=rep(0,4*nr+4);
  for(ir in 1:nr){
    if(ncase==1){
      u0[ir]       =4;
      u0[ir+nr]  =464;
```

```
      u0[ir+2*nr]=227;
      u0[ir+3*nr]= 42;
    }
    if(ncase==2){
      u0[ir]        =4*exp(-25*r[ir]^2);
      u0[ir+nr]   =464*exp(-25*r[ir]^2);
      u0[ir+2*nr]=227*exp(-25*r[ir]^2);
      u0[ir+3*nr]= 42*exp(-25*r[ir]^2);
    }
  }
  u0[4*nr+1]=0;
  u0[4*nr+2]=0;
  u0[4*nr+3]=0;
  u0[4*nr+4]=0;
  ncall=0;
```

$M_p^0 = 0, T_{Cp}^0 = 0, N_p^0 = 0, T_{Rp}^0 = 0$ in ICs (3.3).

- The peripheral variables $M_p(t), T_{Cp}, N_p(t), T_{Rp}(t)$ from the integration of eqs. (3.2) are retrieved from the solution matrix out returned by lsodes [4].

```
#
# Arrays for plotting numerical solution
  M=matrix(0,nrow=nr,ncol=nout);
  TC=matrix(0,nrow=nr,ncol=nout);
  N=matrix(0,nrow=nr,ncol=nout);
  TR=matrix(0,nrow=nr,ncol=nout);
  Mp=rep(0,nout);
  TCp=rep(0,nout);
  Np=rep(0,nout);
  TRp=rep(0,nout);
  for(it in 1:nout){
  for(ir in 1:nr){
    M[ir,it]=out[it,ir+1];
    TC[ir,it]=out[it,ir+nr+1];
    N[ir,it]=out[it,ir+2*nr+1];
    TR[ir,it]=out[it,ir+3*nr+1];
  }
  Mp[it]=out[it,4*nr+2];
  TCp[it]=out[it,4*nr+3];
  Np[it]=out[it,4*nr+4];
  TRp[it]=out[it,4*nr+5];
  }
```

$M_p(t), T_{Cp}, N_p(t), T_{Rp}(t)$ are the final four ODE solutions in matrix out. Matrix out has the row dimension nout=41 and column dimension 4*nr+5 = 4*21+4+1 = 89 as confirmed in the numerical output discussed subsequently. The offset +1 is required since the first element of each solution vector is the value of t.

- Plotting of the peripheral variables is added to the end of the main program.
  par(mfrow=c(2,2)); is used to give a 2×2 matrix of four plots on one page.

Listing 3.1: Excerpts from the main program for eqs. (2.1), (2.2), (3.1) through (3.3)

```
#
# Plot ODE solutions
#
# 2 x 2 matrix of plots
  par(mfrow=c(2,2));
#
# Mp(t)
  plot(tout,Mp,xlab="time (days)",ylab="Mp(t)",
    xlim=c(t0,tf),main="",type="l",lwd=2,
    col="black");
#
# TCp(t)
  plot(tout,TCp,xlab="time (days)",ylab="TCp(t)",
    xlim=c(t0,tf),main="",type="l",lwd=2,
    col="black");
#
# Np(t)
  plot(tout,Np,xlab="time (days)",ylab="Np(t)",
    xlim=c(t0,tf),main="",type="l",lwd=2,
    col="black");
#
# TRp(t)
  plot(tout,TRp,xlab="time (days)",ylab="TRp(t)",
    xlim=c(t0,tf),main="",type="l",lwd=2,
    col="black");
```

The ODE/MOL routine pde1a called by lsodes follows.

(3.1.2) ODE/MOL routine

The following ODE/PDE routine of Listing 3.2 includes the ODEs for the peripheral dependent variables of eqs. (3.2).

Listing 3.2: ODE/MOL routine pde1a for eqs. (2.1), (2.2), (3.1)
through (3.3)

```
pde1a=function(t,u,parm){
#
# Function pde1a computes the t derivative
# vector of M(r,t), TR(r,t), N(r,t), TR(r,t),
# Mp(t), TRp(t), Np(t), TRp(t)
#
# One vector to four vectors, four scalars
  M=rep(0,nr);
  TC=rep(0,nr);
  N=rep(0,nr);
  TR=rep(0,nr);
  for(ir in 1:nr){
    M[ir]=u[ir];
    TC[ir]=u[ir+nr];
    N[ir]=u[ir+2*nr];
    TR[ir]=u[ir+3*nr];
  }
  Mp=u[4*nr+1];
  TCp=u[4*nr+2];
  Np=u[4*nr+3];
  TRp=u[4*nr+4];
#
# Mr,TCr,Nr,TRr
  Mr=dss004(rl,ru,nr, M);
  TCr=dss004(rl,ru,nr,TC);
  Nr=dss004(rl,ru,nr, N);
  TRr=dss004(rl,ru,nr,TR);
#
# BCs
  Mr[1]=0;   Mr[nr]= kM*( Mp- M[nr]);
 TCr[1]=0;  TCr[nr]=kTC*(TCp-TC[nr]);
  Nr[1]=0;   Nr[nr]= kN*( Np- N[nr]);
 TRr[1]=0;  TRr[nr]=kTR*(TRp-TR[nr]);
#
# Mrr,TCrr,Nrr,TRrr
  nl=2;nu=2;
```

(*Continued*)

Listing 3.2 (Continued): ODE/MOL routine `pde1a` **for eqs. (2.1), (2.2), (3.1) through (3.3)**

```
  Mrr=dss044(rl,ru,nr, M, Mr,nl,nu);
 TCrr=dss044(rl,ru,nr,TC,TCr,nl,nu);
  Nrr=dss044(rl,ru,nr, N, Nr,nl,nu);
 TRrr=dss044(rl,ru,nr,TR,TRr,nl,nu);
#
# PDEs
  Mt=rep(0,nr);
 TCt=rep(0,nr);
  Nt=rep(0,nr);
 TRt=rep(0,nr);
 for(ir in 1:nr){
   if(ir==1){
     Mt[ir]=DM*2*Mrr[ir]+
            sM+rM*(1-M[ir]/KM)*M[ir]-
            delM*(1+(aNM*N[ir]/(bNM+N[ir])+
            aCM*TC[ir]/(bCM+TC[ir])+
            aCNM*N[ir]/(bNM+N[ir])*TC[ir]/(bCM+TC[ir]))*
            (1-aMM*M[ir]/(bMM+M[ir])-
            aRM*TR[ir]/(bRM+TR[ir])))*M[ir];
    TCt[ir]=DTC*2*TCrr[ir]+
            rC*(1-TC[ir]/KC)*(1+aMC*M[ir]/(bMC+M[ir])+
            aNC*TR[ir]/(bRM+TR[ir]))*TC[ir]-delC*TC[ir];
     Nt[ir]=DN*2*Nrr[ir]+
            sN+rN*(1-N[ir]/KN)*(1+aCN*TC[ir]/(bCN+TC[ir]))*
            N[ir]-delN*N[ir];
    TRt[ir]=DTR*2*TRrr[ir]+
            rR*(1-TR[ir]/KR)*(1+aMR*M[ir]/(bMR+M[ir]))*
            TR[ir]-delR*TR[ir];
   }
   if(ir>1){
     Mt[ir]=DM*(Mrr[ir]+(1/r[ir])*Mr[ir])+
            sM+rM*(1-M[ir]/KM)*M[ir]-
            delM*(1+(aNM*N[ir]/(bNM+N[ir])+
            aCM*TC[ir]/(bCM+TC[ir])+
            aCNM*N[ir]/(bNM+N[ir])*TC[ir]/(bCM+TC[ir]))*
            (1-aMM*M[ir]/(bMM+M[ir])-
            aRM*TR[ir]/(bRM+TR[ir])))*M[ir];
```

(Continued)

Listing 3.2 (Continued): ODE/MOL routine pde1a for eqs. (2.1), (2.2), (3.1) through (3.3)

```
      TCt[ir]=DTC*(TCrr[ir]+(1/r[ir])*TCr[ir])+
              rC*(1-TC[ir]/KC)*(1+aMC*M[ir]/(bMC+M[ir])+
              aNC*TR[ir]/(bRM+TR[ir]))*TC[ir]-delC*TC[ir];
      Nt[ir]=DN*(Nrr[ir]+(1/r[ir])*Nr[ir])+
              sN+rN*(1-N[ir]/KN)*(1+aCN*TC[ir]/(bCN+TC[ir]))*
              N[ir]-delN*N[ir];
      TRt[ir]=DTR*(TRrr[ir]+(1/r[ir])*TRr[ir])+
              rR*(1-TR[ir]/KR)*(1+aMR*M[ir]/(bMR+M[ir]))*
              TR[ir]-delR*TR[ir];
    }
  }
#
# Peripheral ODEs
  Mpt= -kM*( Mp- M[nr]);
 TCpt=-kTC*(TCp-TC[nr]);
  Npt= -kN*( Np- N[nr]);
 TRpt=-kTR*(TRp-TR[nr]);
#
# t derivative vector
  ut=rep(0,4*nr+4);
  for(ir in 1:nr){
    ut[ir]     = Mt[ir];
    ut[ir+nr]  =TCt[ir];
    ut[ir+2*nr]= Nt[ir];
    ut[ir+3*nr]=TRt[ir];
  }
    ut[4*nr+1]= Mpt;
    ut[4*nr+2]=TCpt;
    ut[4*nr+3]= Npt;
    ut[4*nr+4]=TRpt;
#
# Increment calls to pde1a
  ncall<<-ncall+1;
#
# Return derivative vector
  return(list(c(ut)));
}
```

We can note the following details about pde1a (with some duplication of the explanation of pde1a in Listing 2.2).

- The function is defined.

```
pde1a=function(t,u,parm){
#
# Function pde1a computes the t derivative
# vector of M(r,t), TR(r,t), N(r,t), TR(r,t),
# Mp(t), TRp(t), Np(t), TRp(t)
```

t is the current value of t in eqs. (2.1), (3.2). u is the current numerical solution to eqs. (2.1), (3.2) in the order of the initial condition (IC) vector u0 defined in the main program of Listing 3.1. parm is an argument to pass parameters to pde1a (unused, but required in the argument list). The MOL approximations of the partial derivatives in t of eqs. (2.1) $\frac{\partial M(r,t)}{\partial t}$, $\frac{\partial T_C(r,t)}{\partial t}$, $\frac{\partial N(r,t)}{\partial t}$, $\frac{\partial T_R(r,t)}{\partial t}$ and the ordinary derivatives in t of eqs. (3.2) $\frac{dM_p(t)}{dt}$, $\frac{dT_{Cp}(t)}{dt}$, $\frac{dN_p(t)}{dt}$, $\frac{dT_{Rp}(t)}{dt}$ are calculated and returned to lsodes as explained subsequently.
- The dependent variable vector u is placed in four vectors, M,TC,N,TR, for eqs. (2.1) and four scalars, Np,TCp,Np,TRp, for eqs. (3.2) to facilitate the programming.

```
#
# One vector to four vectors, four scalars
  M=rep(0,nr);
  TC=rep(0,nr);
  N=rep(0,nr);
  TR=rep(0,nr);
  for(ir in 1:nr){
    M[ir]=u[ir];
    TC[ir]=u[ir+nr];
    N[ir]=u[ir+2*nr];
    TR[ir]=u[ir+3*nr];
  }
  Mp=u[4*nr+1];
  TCp=u[4*nr+2];
  Np=u[4*nr+3];
  TRp=u[4*nr+4];
```

- The first derivatives in eqs. (2.1) $\frac{\partial M(r,t)}{\partial r}$, $\frac{\partial T_C(r,t)}{\partial r}$, $\frac{\partial N(r,t)}{\partial r}$, $\frac{\partial T_R(r,t)}{\partial r}$ are computed with dss004. The arguments of dss004 are explained in Appendix A1.
- BCs (3.1) are programmed.

```
#
# BCs
  Mr[1]=0;   Mr[nr]= kM*( Mp- M[nr]);
 TCr[1]=0;  TCr[nr]=kTC*(TCp-TC[nr]);
  Nr[1]=0;   Nr[nr]= kN*( Np- N[nr]);
 TRr[1]=0;  TRr[nr]=kTR*(TRp-TR[nr]);
```

BCs (3.1-1,3,5,7) are programmed at r grid point 1. The Robin BCs of eqs. (3.1-2,4,6,8) are programmed at grid point nr.

- The second derivatives in eqs. (2.1) $\frac{\partial^2 M(r,t)}{\partial r^2}$, $\frac{\partial^2 T_C(r,t)}{\partial r^2}$, $\frac{\partial^2 N(r,t)}{\partial r^2}$, $\frac{\partial^2 T_R(r,t)}{\partial r^2}$ are computed with dss044. The arguments of dss044 are explained in Appendix A1. nl=2,nu=2 specify Neumann BCs at $r = r_l = 0, r = r_u = 1$, respectively, but this also includes the Robin BCs of eqs. (3.1-2,4,6,8) since the first derivatives at $r = r_u$ are computed.

```
#
# Mrr,TCrr,Nrr,TRrr
  nl=2;nu=2;
    Mrr=dss044(rl,ru,nr, M, Mr,nl,nu);
   TCrr=dss044(rl,ru,nr,TC,TCr,nl,nu);
    Nrr=dss044(rl,ru,nr, N, Nr,nl,nu);
   TRrr=dss044(rl,ru,nr,TR,TRr,nl,nu);
```

- Equation (2.1) are programmed within the MOL framework (as previously in Listing 2.2).

```
#
# PDEs
  Mt=rep(0,nr);
 TCt=rep(0,nr);
  Nt=rep(0,nr);
 TRt=rep(0,nr);
 for(ir in 1:nr){
   if(ir==1){
     Mt[ir]=DM*2*Mrr[ir]+
            sM+rM*(1-M[ir]/KM)*M[ir]-
            delM*(1+(aNM*N[ir]/(bNM+N[ir])+
            aCM*TC[ir]/(bCM+TC[ir])+
            aCNM*N[ir]/(bNM+N[ir])*TC[ir]/(bCM+TC[ir]))*
```

```
                        (1-aMM*M[ir]/(bMM+M[ir])-
                        aRM*TR[ir]/(bRM+TR[ir])))*M[ir];
        TCt[ir]=DTC*2*TCrr[ir]+
                        rC*(1-TC[ir]/KC)*(1+aMC*M[ir]/(bMC+M[ir])+
                        aNC*TR[ir]/(bRM+TR[ir]))*TC[ir]-delC*TC[ir];
         Nt[ir]=DN*2*Nrr[ir]+
                        sN+rN*(1-N[ir]/KN)*(1+aCN*TC[ir]/(bCN+
                        TC[ir]))*N[ir]-delN*N[ir];
        TRt[ir]=DTR*2*TRrr[ir]+
                        rR*(1-TR[ir]/KR)*(1+aMR*M[ir]/(bMR+M[ir]))*
                        TR[ir]-delR*TR[ir];
        }
        if(ir>1){
          Mt[ir]=DM*(Mrr[ir]+(1/r[ir])*Mr[ir])+
                        sM+rM*(1-M[ir]/KM)*M[ir]-
                        delM*(1+(aNM*N[ir]/(bNM+N[ir])+
                        aCM*TC[ir]/(bCM+TC[ir])+
                        aCNM*N[ir]/(bNM+N[ir])*TC[ir]/(bCM+TC[ir]))*
                        (1-aMM*M[ir]/(bMM+M[ir])-
                        aRM*TR[ir]/(bRM+TR[ir])))*M[ir];
        TCt[ir]=DTC*(TCrr[ir]+(1/r[ir])*TCr[ir])+
                        rC*(1-TC[ir]/KC)*(1+aMC*M[ir]/(bMC+M[ir])+
                        aNC*TR[ir]/(bRM+TR[ir]))*TC[ir]-delC*TC[ir];
         Nt[ir]=DN*(Nrr[ir]+(1/r[ir])*Nr[ir])+
                        sN+rN*(1-N[ir]/KN)*(1+aCN*TC[ir]/(bCN+
                        TC[ir]))*N[ir]-delN*N[ir];
        TRt[ir]=DTR*(TRrr[ir]+(1/r[ir])*TRr[ir])+
                        rR*(1-TR[ir]/KR)*(1+aMR*M[ir]/(bMR+M[ir]))*
                        TR[ir]-delR*TR[ir];
        }
      }
#
# Peripheral ODEs
   Mpt= -kM*( Mp- M[nr]);
  TCpt=-kTC*(TCp-TC[nr]);
   Npt= -kN*( Np- N[nr]);
  TRpt=-kTR*(TRp-TR[nr]);
```

The ODEs of eqs. (3.2) are added at the end to give a total of $4 \times 21 + 4 = 4(21) + 4 = 88$ ordinary derivatives in t.

- The 4*nr+4 $= 88$ derivatives in t are placed in a single vector, ut, for return to lsodes.

```
#
# t derivative vector
  ut=rep(0,4*nr+4);
  for(ir in 1:nr){
    ut[ir]      = Mt[ir];
    ut[ir+nr]   =TCt[ir];
    ut[ir+2*nr]= Nt[ir];
    ut[ir+3*nr]=TRt[ir];
  }
    ut[4*nr+1]= Mpt;
    ut[4*nr+2]=TCpt;
    ut[4*nr+3]= Npt;
    ut[4*nr+4]=TRpt;
```

- The number of calls to pde1a is incremented and returned to the main program by <<-.

```
#
# Increment calls to pde1a
  ncall<<-ncall+1;
```

- The derivative vector of length 88 is returned to lsodes as a list as required by lsodes. c is the R vector utility.

```
#
# Return derivative vector
  return(list(c(ut)));
}
```

The final } concludes pde1a.

This concludes the programming of the R routines. The numerical and graphical output is considered next.

(3.1.3) Numerical, graphical output

Abbreviated numerical for `ncase=1` (set in the main programs of Listings 2.1, 3.1) follows.

Table 3.1: Abbreviated output for `ncase=1`

[1] 41

[1] 89

t	r	M(t)	TC(t)	N(t)	TR(t)
0.00	0.00	4.000	464.000	227.000	42.000
0.00	0.25	4.000	464.000	227.000	42.000
0.00	0.50	4.000	464.000	227.000	42.000
0.00	0.75	4.000	464.000	227.000	42.000
0.00	1.00	4.000	464.000	227.000	42.000

t		Mp(t)	TCp(t)	Np(t)	TRp(t)
0.00		0.000	0.000	0.000	0.000

t	r	M(t)	TC(t)	N(t)	TR(t)
100.00	0.00	4.570	533.274	272.048	46.922
100.00	0.25	4.570	533.274	272.048	46.922
100.00	0.50	4.570	533.274	272.048	46.922
100.00	0.75	4.570	533.268	272.047	46.922
100.00	1.00	4.568	533.227	272.034	46.919

t		Mp(t)	TCp(t)	Np(t)	TRp(t)
100.00		4.564	533.093	271.973	46.912

.
.
.

Output for t = 200,...,900 removed

.
.
.

t	r	M(t)	TC(t)	N(t)	TR(t)
1000.00	0.00	5.221	545.304	274.167	47.898
1000.00	0.25	5.221	545.304	274.167	47.898
1000.00	0.50	5.221	545.304	274.167	47.898
1000.00	0.75	5.221	545.304	274.167	47.898
1000.00	1.00	5.221	545.304	274.167	47.898

t		Mp(t)	TCp(t)	Np(t)	TRp(t)
1000.00		5.221	545.304	274.167	47.898

ncall =   303

We can note the following details about this output.

- 41 output points in t (from nout=41 in the main program of Listings 2.1 and 3.1) as the first dimension of the solution matrix out from lsodes.
- The solution matrix out returned by lsodes has 89 elements as a second dimension. The first element is the value of t. Elements 2 to 85 in out are $M(r,t)$, $T_C(r,t)$, $N(r,t)$, $T_R(r,t)$ for eqs. (2.1). Elements 86 to 89 in out are $M_p(r,t)$, $T_{Cp}(r,t)$, $N_p(r,t)$, $T_{Rp}(r,t)$ for eqs. (3.2).
- The solution is displayed for $t = 0, 100, ..., 1000$ and $r = 0, 0.05, ..., 1$ as programmed in Listings 2.1, 3.1 (every fourth value of t and every fifth value of r, as discussed previously).
- ICs (2.2), (3.3) ($t = 0$) are confirmed. This check is important since if the ICs are not correct, the subsequent solution will also not be correct. Note in particular the constant values in r (from the ICs with ncase=1).
- The solutions remain invariant (constant) in r which is expected from the homogeneous Neumann and Robin BCs (3.1) (the RHS mass transfer term in BCs (3.1-2,4,6,8) is zero). This may seem like a trivial case, but it is worth considering since a variation of the solutions in r would indicate a programming error.
- The PDE solutions agree with the ODE solutions of Chapter 1, Table 1.4, and the PDE solutions of Chapter 2, Table 2.1. For example, at $t = 1000$

Table 1.4

t	M(t)	TC(t)	N(t)	TR(t)
1000.00	5.221	545.304	274.167	47.898

Table 2.1

t	r	M(t)	TC(t)	N(t)	TR(t)
1000.00	0.00	5.221	545.304	274.167	47.898
1000.00	0.25	5.221	545.304	274.167	47.898
1000.00	0.50	5.221	545.304	274.167	47.898
1000.00	0.75	5.221	545.304	274.167	47.898
1000.00	1.00	5.221	545.304	274.167	47.898

Table 3.1

t	r	M(t)	TC(t)	N(t)	TR(t)
1000.00	0.00	5.221	545.304	274.167	47.898
1000.00	0.25	5.221	545.304	274.167	47.898
1000.00	0.50	5.221	545.304	274.167	47.898
1000.00	0.75	5.221	545.304	274.167	47.898
1000.00	1.00	5.221	545.304	274.167	47.898

t		Mp(t)	TCp(t)	Np(t)	TRp(t)
1000.00		5.221	545.304	274.167	47.898

- The computational effort is modest, `ncall` = 303, so that `lsodes` efficiently computed a solution to eqs. (2.1), (3.2).

The graphical output follows (six figures with `matplot`, `persp` are not included since they are similar to Figures 3.1-3 through 3.1-8).

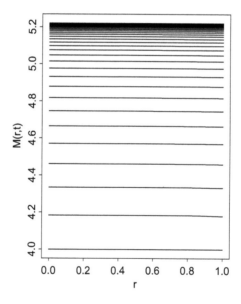

Figure 3.1-1: Numerical solution $M(r,t)$ from eq. (2.1-1), `ncase=1`, `matplot`.

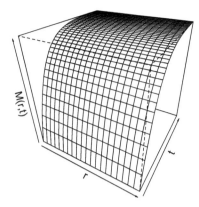

Figure 3.1-2: Numerical solution $M(r,t)$ from eq. (2.1-1), `ncase=1`, `persp`.

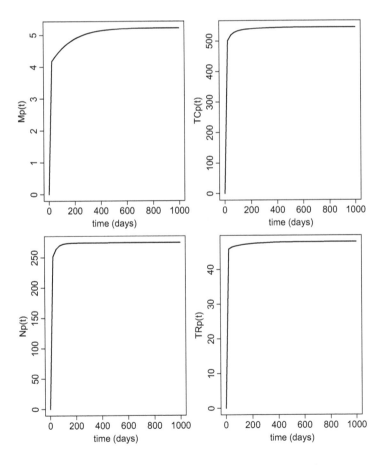

Figure 3.1-9: Numerical solutions $M_p(t)$ to $T_{Rp}(t)$ from eqs. (3.2), `ncase=1`.

We can note that ICs (2.2) and (3.3) are confirmed, and the equilibrium solutions of eqs. (3.2) as $t \to 1000$ as listed in Table 3.1

For ncase=2, the abbreviated numerical output is in Table 3.2.

Table 3.2: Abbreviated output for ncase=2

[1] 41

[1] 89

t	r	M(t)	TC(t)	N(t)	TR(t)
0.00	0.00	4.000	464.000	227.000	42.000
0.00	0.25	0.838	97.260	47.582	8.804
0.00	0.50	0.008	0.896	0.438	0.081
0.00	0.75	0.000	0.000	0.000	0.000
0.00	1.00	0.000	0.000	0.000	0.000

t		Mp(t)	TCp(t)	Np(t)	TRp(t)
0.00		0.000	0.000	0.000	0.000

t	r	M(t)	TC(t)	N(t)	TR(t)
100.00	0.00	3.195	469.800	254.286	43.768
100.00	0.25	1.903	277.228	182.057	36.203
100.00	0.50	0.477	12.900	26.128	5.791
100.00	0.75	0.238	0.088	7.114	0.048
100.00	1.00	0.233	0.001	6.821	0.000

t		Mp(t)	TCp(t)	Np(t)	TRp(t)
100.00		0.228	0.001	6.695	0.000

```
                          .                 .
                          .                 .
                          .                 .
            Output for t = 200,...,900 removed
                          .                 .
                          .                 .
                          .                 .
```

t	r	M(t)	TC(t)	N(t)	TR(t)
1000.00	0.00	5.201	545.026	274.150	47.872
1000.00	0.25	5.202	545.038	274.151	47.873
1000.00	0.50	5.205	545.080	274.153	47.877
1000.00	0.75	5.209	545.136	274.157	47.882
1000.00	1.00	5.211	545.162	274.158	47.885

t		Mp(t)	TCp(t)	Np(t)	TRp(t)
1000.00		5.211	545.161	274.158	47.884

ncall =   429

We can note the following details about this output.

- Radial profiles in r develop from the Gaussian function ICs (eqs. (2.2)).
- The solutions for the four dependent variable components (Table 1.1) approach the same equilibrium solutions as for ncase=1.
- The computational effort is modest, ncall = 429.

The graphical output in Figure 3.2 confirms the properties of the numerical solutions, in particular, (1) the fronts moving left to right in r resulting from the radial diffusion and BCs (3.1-2,4,6,8), (2) the approach to the same equilibrium solutions as for ncase=1, and (3) the agreement of the PDE solutions (for eqs. (2.1)) and the ODE solutions (for eqs. (3.2)).

The moving front solutions in response to the Gaussian ICs and the approach to equilibrium solutions is clear in the graphical output that follows.

Figures 3.2-1 through 3.2-8 indicate the Gaussian ICs and the equilibrium solutions as $t \to 1000$.

The approach of the ODE solutions of eqs. (3.2) (Figure 3.2-9) is similar to the solutions in Figure 3.1-9, but with a lag in t resulting from the movement of the PDE Gaussian ICs from left to right toward the outer boundary at $r = r_u$.

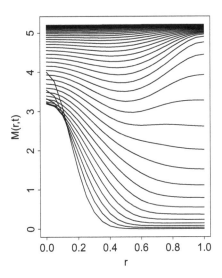

Figure 3.2-1: Numerical solution $M(r,t)$ from eq. (2.1-1), ncase=2, matplot.

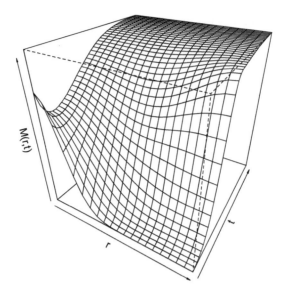

Figure 3.2-2: Numerical solution $M(r, t)$ from eq. (2.1-1), `ncase=2`, `persp`.

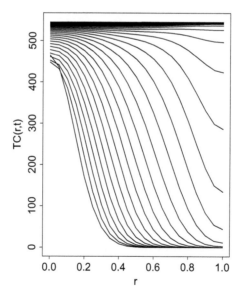

Figure 3.2-3: Numerical solution $T_C(r, t)$ from eq. (2.1-2), `ncase=2`, `matplot`.

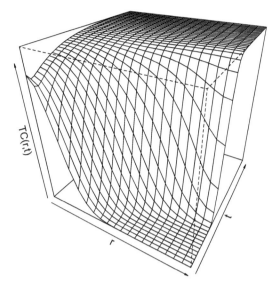

Figure 3.2-4: Numerical solution $T_C(r, t)$ from eq. (2.1-2), `ncase=2`, `persp`.

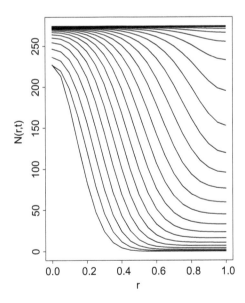

Figure 3.2-5: Numerical solution $N(r, t)$ from eq. (2.1-3), `ncase=2`, `matplot`.

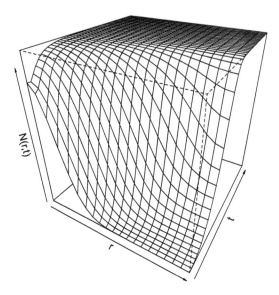

Figure 3.2-6: Numerical solution $M(r, t)$ from eq. (2.1-3), ncase=2, persp.

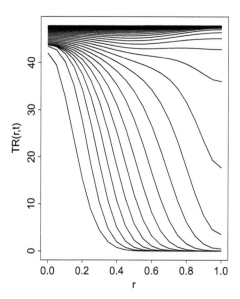

Figure 3.2-7: Numerical solution $T_R(r, t)$ from eq. (2.1-4), ncase=2, matplot.

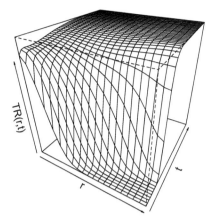

Figure 3.2-8: Numerical solution $T_R(r, t)$ from eq. (2.1-4), `ncase=2`, `persp`.

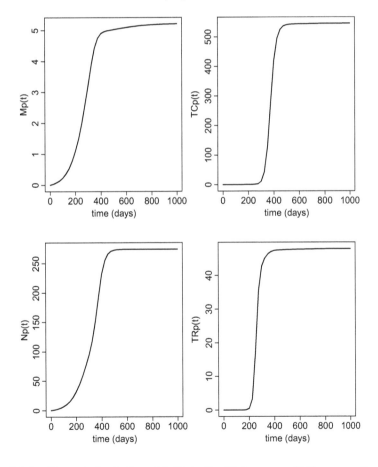

Figure 3.2-9: Numerical solutions $M_p(t)$ to $T_{Rp}(t)$ from eqs. (3.2), `ncase=2`.

(3.2)　Summary and conclusions

The MOL implementation of the ODE/PDE model of eqs. (2.1), (2.2), (3.1), (3.2), (3.3) is in the R routines of Listings 2.1, 3.1, 3.2. In particular, the ODE solutions for the dependent variable components (Table 3.2) in the peripheral blood follow the PDE solutions for the bone marrow.

As another example of the ODE/PDE model, the effect of variable diffusivities in the bone marrow is considered in Chapter 4.

References

1. Gallaher, J., et al. (2018), A Mathematical Model for TumorImmune Dynamics in Multiple Myeloma, *Understanding Complex Biological Systems with Mathematics*, A. Radunskaya, R. Segal, and B. Shtylla (eds.), Association for Women in Mathematics Series, vol. 14, Chapter 5, pp. 89–122, Springer, Cham.
2. Gallaher, J., et al. (2018), Methods for determining key components in a mathematical model for tumor-immune dynamics in multiple myeloma, *Journal of Theoretical Biology*, **458**, pp. 31–46.
3. Schiesser, W.E. (2016), *Method of Lines PDE Analysis in Biomedical Science and Engineering*, John Wiley & Sons, Hoboken, NJ.
4. Soetaert, K., J. Cash, and F. Mazzia (2012), *Solving Differential Equations in R*, Springer-Verlag, Heidelberg, Germany.

4 ODE/PDE Model Parameter Analysis

(4) Introduction

The ODE/PDE model of Chapter 3 can be used for computer-based experimentation, which, for example, can include variation of the model parameters and structure. In this chapter, the diffusivities are varied radially to reflect the decrease in the permeability of the bone marrow with increasing r, with small diffusivities for the hard bone near the outer boundary at $r = r_u$.

(4.1) ODE/PDE model with variable diffusivity

If the diffusivities in eqs. (2.1) are functions of r, then these terms require expansion (additional differentiation) in r. For example, for eq. (2.1-1), the radial diffusion term is (with $D_M(r)$)

$$\frac{1}{r}\frac{\partial\left(rD_M(r)\dfrac{\partial M(r,t)}{\partial r}\right)}{\partial r}$$

$$= D_M(r)\frac{\partial^2 M(r,t)}{\partial r^2} + \frac{dD_M(r)}{dr}\frac{\partial M(r,t)}{\partial r} + \frac{1}{r}D_M(r)\frac{\partial M(r,t)}{\partial r} \qquad (4.1\text{-}1)$$

The variable diffusivity $D_M(r)$ is expressed as the constant diffusivity D_M multiplied by a function of r, $D_M D(r)$, where, for example, $D(r)$ is a piecewise linear function in r.

$$D(r) = \begin{cases} 1, & r_l \leq r < r_1 \\[2mm] 1 - \dfrac{0.9}{(r_2 - r_1)}(r - r_1), & r_1 \leq r < r_2 \\[2mm] 0.1, & r_2 \leq r \leq r_u \end{cases} \qquad (4.1\text{-}2)$$

r_1, r_2 are parameters (constants) that define the sections of $D(r)$ (with linear variations in r for $r_l \leq r \leq r_u$).

Equation (4.1-1) includes the derivative of $D_M(r)$, $\dfrac{dD_M(r)}{dr}$, or $D_M \dfrac{dD(r)}{dr}$, with (from eq. (4.1-2))

$$\frac{dD(r)}{dr} = \begin{cases} 0, & r_l \leq r < r_1 \\[2mm] -\dfrac{0.9}{(r_2 - r_1)}, & r_1 \leq r < r_2 \\[2mm] 0, & r_2 \leq r \leq r_u \end{cases} \qquad (4.1\text{-}3)$$

The functions of eqs. (4.1-2,3), $D(r)$, $\dfrac{dD(r)}{dr}$, are implemented in functions Dr, Drr, respectively, in the subsequent R programming. $D(r)$ consists of three parts, (1) a left section, starting at $r = r_l$, ending at $r = r_1$, with a constant value of 1, (2) a middle section, starting at $r = r_1$, ending at $r = r_2$, and linearly decreasing from 1 to 0.1, and (3) a right section starting at $r = r_2$, ending at $r = r_u$, with a constant value of 0.1. $\dfrac{dD(r)}{dr}$ has the corresponding derivative values. For example, the diffusivity $D_M(r)$ decreases from D_M to $0.1D_M$ in approaching the right outer boundary at $r = r_u$.

With the use of the variable diffusivity of eqs. (4.1), eqs. (2.1) and (3.2) are modified to eqs. (4.2).

$$\frac{\partial M}{\partial t} = D_M D(r) \left(\frac{\partial^2 M}{\partial r^2} + \frac{1}{r} \frac{\partial M}{\partial r} \right) + D_M \frac{dD(r)}{dr} \frac{\partial M}{\partial r} + s_M + r_M \left(1 - \frac{M}{K_M} \right) M$$

$$- \delta_M \left[1 + \left(\frac{a_{NM} N}{b_{NM} + N} + \frac{a_{CM} T_C}{b_{CM} + T_C} + a_{CNM} \frac{N}{b_{NM} + N} \cdot \frac{T_C}{b_{CM} + T_C} \right) \cdot \right.$$

$$\left. \left(1 - \frac{a_{MM} M}{b_{MM} + M} - \frac{a_{RM} T_R}{b_{RM} + T_R} \right) \right] \cdot M \qquad (4.2\text{-}1)$$

$$\frac{\partial T_C}{\partial t} = D_{T_C} D(r) \left(\frac{\partial^2 T_C}{\partial r^2} + \frac{1}{r} \frac{\partial T_C}{\partial r} \right) + D_{T_C} \frac{dD(r)}{dr} \frac{\partial T_C}{\partial r}$$

$$+ r_C \left(1 - \frac{T_C}{K_C} \right) \left(1 + \frac{a_{MC} M}{b_{MC} + M} + \frac{a_{NC} N}{b_{NC} + N} \right) T_C - \delta_C T_C \qquad (4.2\text{-}2)$$

$$\frac{\partial N}{\partial t} = D_N D(r) \left(\frac{\partial^2 N}{\partial r^2} + \frac{1}{r} \frac{\partial N}{\partial r} \right) + D_N \frac{dD(r)}{dr} \frac{\partial N}{\partial r}$$

$$+ s_N + r_N \left(1 - \frac{N}{K_N} \right) \left(1 + \frac{a_{CN} T_C}{b_{CN} + T_C} \right) N - \delta_N N \qquad (4.2\text{-}3)$$

$$\frac{\partial T_R}{\partial t} = D_{T_C} D(r) \left(\frac{\partial^2 T_R}{\partial r^2} + \frac{1}{r} \frac{\partial T_C}{\partial r} \right) + D_{T_R} \frac{dD(r)}{dr} \frac{\partial T_R}{\partial r}$$

$$+r_R\left(1 - \frac{T_R}{K_R}\right)\left(1 + \frac{a_{MR}M}{b_{MR} + M}\right)T_R - \delta_R T_R \qquad (4.2\text{-}4)$$

$$\frac{dM_p}{dt} = k_M(M_p(t) - M(r = r_u, t)) \qquad (4.2\text{-}5)$$

$$\frac{dT_{Cp}}{dt} = k_{T_C}(T_{Cp}(t) - T_C(r = r_u, t)) \qquad (4.2\text{-}6)$$

$$\frac{dN_p}{dt} = k_N(N_p(t) - N(r = r_u, t)) \qquad (4.2\text{-}7)$$

$$\frac{dT_{Rp}}{dt} = k_{T_R}(T_{Rp}(t) - T_R(r = r_u, t)) \qquad (4.2\text{-}8)$$

Equations (4.2) are first order in t and require an IC for each equation.

$$M(t = 0) = M^0 = 4 \qquad (4.3\text{-}1)$$

$$T_C(t = 0) = T_C^0 = 464 \qquad (4.3\text{-}2)$$

$$N(t = 0) = N^0 = 227 \qquad (4.3\text{-}3)$$

$$T_R(t = 0) = T_R^0 = 42 \qquad (4.3\text{-}4)$$

$$M_p(t = 0) = M_p^0 = 0 \qquad (4.3\text{-}5)$$

$$T_{Cp}(t = 0) = T_{Cp}^0 = 0 \qquad (4.3\text{-}6)$$

$$N_p(t = 0) = N_p^0 = 0 \qquad (4.3\text{-}7)$$

$$T_{Rp}(t = 0) = T_{Rp}^0 = 0 \qquad (4.3\text{-}8)$$

BCs (3.1) are used again for eqs. (4.2-1,2,3,4).

$$\frac{\partial M(r = r_l, t)}{\partial r} = 0; \quad \frac{\partial M(r = r_u, t)}{\partial r} = k_M(M_p(t) - M(r = r_u, t)) \quad (4.4\text{-}1,2)$$

$$\frac{\partial T_C(r = r_l, t)}{\partial r} = 0; \quad \frac{\partial T_C(r = r_u, t)}{\partial r} = k_{T_C}(T_{Cp}(t) - T_C(r = r_u, t)) \quad (4.4\text{-}3,4)$$

$$\frac{\partial N(r = r_l, t)}{\partial r} = 0; \quad \frac{\partial N(r = r_u, t)}{\partial r} = k_N(N_p(t) - N(r = r_u, t)) \quad (4.4\text{-}5,6)$$

$$\frac{\partial T_R(r = r_l, t)}{\partial r} = 0; \quad \frac{\partial T_R(r = r_u, t)}{\partial r} = k_{T_R}(T_{Rp}(t) - T_R(r = r_u, t)) \quad (4.4\text{-}7,8)$$

Equations (4.2) through (4.4) constitute the ODE/PDE model with variable diffusivities. The model is implemented in the following R routines.

(4.1.1) Main program

The main programs of Listings 2.1 and 3.1 are used with the following minor changes/additions.

Listing 4.1: Modifications of the main program for eqs. (4.1–4)

- The functions `Dr`, `Drr` are accessed.

```
#
# Access functions for numerical solution
  setwd("f:/multipleMyeloma/chap4");
  source("pde1a.R");
  source("Dr.R");
  source("Drr.R");
  source("dss004.R");
  source("dss044.R");
```

- The points r_1, r_2 in eqs. (4.1-2,3) are defined numerically.

```
#
# Diffusivities (cm^2/days)
  days=60*60*24;
   DM=1.0e-09*days;
  DTC=1.0e-09*days;
   DN=1.0e-09*days;
  DTR=1.0e-09*days;
   r1=0.4;
   r2=0.8;
```

- The number of grid points in r is increased to 51 to improve the spatial resolution (remove gridding effcts in the numerical solution).

```
#
# Spatial grid
  rl=0; ru=1; nr=51; dr=(ru-rl)/(nr-1);
  r=seq(from=rl,to=ru,by=dr);
```

(4.1.2) ODE/PDE routine

The ODE/PDE routine of Listing 4.2 for eqs. (4.2), (4.4) is an extension of the routine of Listing 3.2.

Listing 4.2: ODE/MOL routine pde1a for eqs. (4.1), (4.2), (4.4)

```
pde1a=function(t,u,parm){
#
# Function pde1a computes the t derivative
# vector of M(r,t), TR(r,t), N(r,t), TR(r,t),
# Mp(t), TRp(t), Np(t), TRp(t)
#
# One vector to four vectors, four scalars
  M=rep(0,nr);
 TC=rep(0,nr);
  N=rep(0,nr);
 TR=rep(0,nr);
 for(ir in 1:nr){
    M[ir]=u[ir];
   TC[ir]=u[ir+nr];
    N[ir]=u[ir+2*nr];
   TR[ir]=u[ir+3*nr];
  }
  Mp=u[4*nr+1];
 TCp=u[4*nr+2];
  Np=u[4*nr+3];
 TRp=u[4*nr+4];
#
# Mr,TCr,Nr,TRr
   Mr=dss004(rl,ru,nr, M);
  TCr=dss004(rl,ru,nr,TC);
   Nr=dss004(rl,ru,nr, N);
  TRr=dss004(rl,ru,nr,TR);
#
# BCs
  Mr[1]=0;  Mr[nr]= kM*( Mp- M[nr]);
 TCr[1]=0; TCr[nr]=kTC*(TCp-TC[nr]);
  Nr[1]=0;  Nr[nr]= kN*( Np- N[nr]);
 TRr[1]=0; TRr[nr]=kTR*(TRp-TR[nr]);
```

(Continued)

Listing 4.2 (Continued): ODE/MOL routine pde1a for eqs. (4.1),
(4.2), (4.4)

```
#
# Mrr,TCrr,Nrr,TRrr
  nl=2;nu=2;
  Mrr=dss044(rl,ru,nr, M, Mr,nl,nu);
 TCrr=dss044(rl,ru,nr,TC,TCr,nl,nu);
  Nrr=dss044(rl,ru,nr, N, Nr,nl,nu);
 TRrr=dss044(rl,ru,nr,TR,TRr,nl,nu);
#
# PDEs
  Mt=rep(0,nr);
 TCt=rep(0,nr);
  Nt=rep(0,nr);
 TRt=rep(0,nr);
  for(ir in 1:nr){
    if(ir==1){
      Mt[ir]=DM*Dr(r[ir])*2*Mrr[ir]+
             DM*Drr(r[ir])*Mr[ir]+
             sM+rM*(1-M[ir]/KM)*M[ir]-
             delM*(1+(aNM*N[ir]/(bNM+N[ir])+
             aCM*TC[ir]/(bCM+TC[ir])+
             aCNM*N[ir]/(bNM+N[ir])*TC[ir]/(bCM+TC[ir]))*
             (1-aMM*M[ir]/(bMM+M[ir])-
             aRM*TR[ir]/(bRM+TR[ir])))*M[ir];
     TCt[ir]=DTC*Dr(r[ir])*2*TCrr[ir]+
             DTC*Drr(r[ir])*TCr[ir]+
             rC*(1-TC[ir]/KC)*(1+aMC*M[ir]/(bMC+M[ir])+
             aNC*TR[ir]/(bRM+TR[ir]))*TC[ir]-delC*TC[ir];
      Nt[ir]=DN*Dr(r[ir])*2*Nrr[ir]+
             DN*Drr(r[ir])*Nr[ir]+
             sN+rN*(1-N[ir]/KN)*(1+aCN*TC[ir]/(bCN+TC[ir]))*
             N[ir]-delN*N[ir];
     TRt[ir]=DTR*Dr(r[ir])*2*TRrr[ir]+
             DTR*Drr(r[ir])*TRr[ir]+
             rR*(1-TR[ir]/KR)*(1+aMR*M[ir]/(bMR+M[ir]))*
             TR[ir]-delR*TR[ir];
    }
```

(Continued)

Listing 4.2 (Continued): ODE/MOL routine pde1a for eqs. (4.1),
(4.2), (4.4)

```
  if(ir>1){
    Mt[ir]=DM*Dr(r[ir])*(Mrr[ir]+(1/r[ir])*Mr[ir])+
           DM*Drr(r[ir])*Mr[ir]+
           sM+rM*(1-M[ir]/KM)*M[ir]-
           delM*(1+(aNM*N[ir]/(bNM+N[ir])+
           aCM*TC[ir]/(bCM+TC[ir])+
           aCNM*N[ir]/(bNM+N[ir])*TC[ir]/(bCM+TC[ir]))*
           (1-aMM*M[ir]/(bMM+M[ir])-
           aRM*TR[ir]/(bRM+TR[ir])))*M[ir];
    TCt[ir]=DTC*Dr(r[ir])*(TCrr[ir]+(1/r[ir])*TCr[ir])+
           DTC*Drr(r[ir])*TCr[ir]+
           rC*(1-TC[ir]/KC)*(1+aMC*M[ir]/(bMC+M[ir])+
           aNC*TR[ir]/(bRM+TR[ir]))*TC[ir]-delC*TC[ir];
    Nt[ir]=DN*Dr(r[ir])*(Nrr[ir]+(1/r[ir])*Nr[ir])+
           DN*Drr(r[ir])*Nr[ir]+
           sN+rN*(1-N[ir]/KN)*(1+aCN*TC[ir]/(bCN+TC[ir]))*
           N[ir]-delN*N[ir];
    TRt[ir]=DTR*Dr(r[ir])*(TRrr[ir]+(1/r[ir])*TRr[ir])+
           DTR*Drr(r[ir])*TRr[ir]+
           rR*(1-TR[ir]/KR)*(1+aMR*M[ir]/(bMR+M[ir]))*
           TR[ir]-delR*TR[ir];
  }
}
#
# Peripheral ODEs
  Mpt= -kM*( Mp- M[nr]);
 TCpt=-kTC*(TCp-TC[nr]);
  Npt= -kN*( Np- N[nr]);
 TRpt=-kTR*(TRp-TR[nr]);
#
# t derivative vector
  ut=rep(0,4*nr+4);
  for(ir in 1:nr){
    ut[ir]     = Mt[ir];
    ut[ir+nr]   =TCt[ir];
    ut[ir+2*nr]= Nt[ir];
    ut[ir+3*nr]=TRt[ir];
  }
```

(Continued)

Listing 4.2 (Continued): ODE/MOL routine pde1a for eqs. (4.1), (4.2), (4.4)

```
    ut[4*nr+1]= Mpt;
    ut[4*nr+2]=TCpt;
    ut[4*nr+3]= Npt;
    ut[4*nr+4]=TRpt;
#
# Increment calls to pde1a
  ncall<<-ncall+1;
#
# Return derivative vector
  return(list(c(ut)));
}
```

We can note the following details about pde1a (with some duplication of the explanation of pde1a in Listings 2.2, 3.2).

- The function is defined.

```
    pde1a=function(t,u,parm){
#
# Function pde1a computes the t derivative
# vector of M(r,t), TR(r,t), N(r,t), TR(r,t),
# Mp(t), TRp(t), Np(t), TRp(t)
```

  t is the current value of t in eqs. (4.2). u is the current numerical solution to eqs. (4.2), ordered as in the initial condition vector u0. parm is an argument to pass parameters to pde1a (unused, but required in the argument list). The MOL approximations of the partial derivatives in t of eqs. (4.2-1,2,3,4) $\frac{\partial M(r,t)}{\partial t}$, $\frac{\partial T_C(r,t)}{\partial t}$, $\frac{\partial N(r,t)}{\partial t}$, $\frac{\partial T_R(r,t)}{\partial t}$ and the ordinary derivatives in t of eqs. (4.2-5,6,7,8) $\frac{dM_p(t)}{dt}$, $\frac{dT_{Cp}(t)}{dt}$, $\frac{dN_p(t)}{dt}$, $\frac{dT_{Rp}(t)}{dt}$ are calculated and returned to lsodes as explained subsequently.

- The dependent variable vector u is placed in four vectors, M,TC,N,TR and four scalars, Mp,Tcp,Np,TRp, for eqs. (4.2) to facilitate the programming.

```
#
# One vector to four vectors, four scalars
    M=rep(0,nr);
    TC=rep(0,nr);
    N=rep(0,nr);
```

```
TR=rep(0,nr);
for(ir in 1:nr){
   M[ir]=u[ir];
  TC[ir]=u[ir+nr];
   N[ir]=u[ir+2*nr];
  TR[ir]=u[ir+3*nr];
}
 Mp=u[4*nr+1];
TCp=u[4*nr+2];
 Np=u[4*nr+3];
TRp=u[4*nr+4];
```

- The first derivatives in eqs. (4.2-1,2,3,4), $\frac{\partial M(r,t)}{\partial r}$, $\frac{\partial T_C(r,t)}{\partial r}$, $\frac{\partial N(r,t)}{\partial r}$, $\frac{\partial T_R(r,t)}{\partial r}$, are computed with dss004. The arguments of dss004 are explained in Appendix A1.

```
#
# Mr,TCr,Nr,TRr
   Mr=dss004(rl,ru,nr, M);
  TCr=dss004(rl,ru,nr,TC);
   Nr=dss004(rl,ru,nr, N);
  TRr=dss004(rl,ru,nr,TR);
```

- BCs (4.4) are programmed.

```
#
# BCs
  Mr[1]=0;  Mr[nr]= kM*( Mp- M[nr]);
 TCr[1]=0; TCr[nr]=kTC*(TCp-TC[nr]);
  Nr[1]=0;  Nr[nr]= kN*( Np- N[nr]);
 TRr[1]=0; TRr[nr]=kTR*(TRp-TR[nr]);
```

BCs (4.4-1,3,5,7) are programmed at r grid point 1. The Robin BCs of eqs. (4.4-2,4,6,8) are programmed at grid point nr.

- The second derivatives in eqs. (4.2-1,2,3,4), $\frac{\partial^2 M(r,t)}{\partial r^2}$, $\frac{\partial^2 T_C(r,t)}{\partial r^2}$, $\frac{\partial^2 N(r,t)}{\partial r^2}$, $\frac{\partial^2 T_R(r,t)}{\partial r^2}$, are computed with dss044. The arguments of dss044 are explained in Appendix A1. nl=2,nu=2 specify Neumann BCs at $r = r_l = 0, r = r_u = 1$, respectively, but this also includes the Robin BCs of eqs. (4.4-2,4,6,8) since the first derivatives at $r = r_u$ are computed.

```
#
# Mrr,TCrr,Nrr,TRrr
  nl=2;nu=2;
  Mrr=dss044(rl,ru,nr, M, Mr,nl,nu);
  TCrr=dss044(rl,ru,nr,TC,TCr,nl,nu);
  Nrr=dss044(rl,ru,nr, N, Nr,nl,nu);
  TRrr=dss044(rl,ru,nr,TR,TRr,nl,nu);
```

- Equations (4.2-1,2,3,4) are programmed within the MOL framework.

```
#
# PDEs
  Mt=rep(0,nr);
  TCt=rep(0,nr);
  Nt=rep(0,nr);
  TRt=rep(0,nr);
  for(ir in 1:nr){
```

For $r = 0$

```
  if(ir==1){
```

- Eq. (4.2-1) is programmed.
```
      Mt[ir]=DM*Dr(r[ir])*2*Mrr[ir]+
             DM*Drr(r[ir])*Mr[ir]+
             sM+rM*(1-M[ir]/KM)*M[ir]-
             delM*(1+(aNM*N[ir]/(bNM+N[ir])+
             aCM*TC[ir]/(bCM+TC[ir])+
             aCNM*N[ir]/(bNM+N[ir])*TC[ir]/(bCM+
             TC[ir]))*(1-aMM*M[ir]/(bMM+M[ir])-
             aRM*TR[ir]/(bRM+TR[ir])))*M[ir];
```
- Eq. (4.2-2) is programmed.
```
      TCt[ir]=DTC*Dr(r[ir])*2*TCrr[ir]+
              DTC*Drr(r[ir])*TCr[ir]+
              rC*(1-TC[ir]/KC)*(1+aMC*M[ir]/(bMC+M[ir])+
              aNC*TR[ir]/(bRM+TR[ir]))*TC[ir]-delC*
              TC[ir];
```
- Eq. (4.2-3) is programmed.
```
      Nt[ir]=DN*Dr(r[ir])*2*Nrr[ir]+
             DN*Drr(r[ir])*Nr[ir]+
             sN+rN*(1-N[ir]/KN)*(1+aCN*TC[ir]/(bCN+
             TC[ir]))*N[ir]-delN*N[ir];
```

− Eq. (4.2-4) is programmed.

```
TRt[ir]=DTR*Dr(r[ir])*2*TRrr[ir]+
        DTR*Drr(r[ir])*TRr[ir]+
        rR*(1-TR[ir]/KR)*(1+aMR*M[ir]/(bMR+M[ir]))*
        TR[ir]-delR*TR[ir];
  }
```

The final } concludes the **for** with $r = 0$.

For $r > 0$

```
if(ir>1){
```

− Eq. (4.2-1) is programmed.

```
Mt[ir]=DM*Dr(r[ir])*(Mrr[ir]+(1/r[ir])*Mr[ir])+
       DM*Drr(r[ir])*Mr[ir]+
       sM+rM*(1-M[ir]/KM)*M[ir]-
       delM*(1+(aNM*N[ir]/(bNM+N[ir])+
       aCM*TC[ir]/(bCM+TC[ir])+
       aCNM*N[ir]/(bNM+N[ir])*TC[ir]/(bCM+
       TC[ir]))*(1-aMM*M[ir]/(bMM+M[ir])-
       aRM*TR[ir]/(bRM+TR[ir])))*M[ir];
```

− Eq. (4.2-2) is programmed.

```
TCt[ir]=DTC*Dr(r[ir])*(TCrr[ir]+(1/r[ir])*TCr[ir])+
        DTC*Drr(r[ir])*TCr[ir]+
        rC*(1-TC[ir]/KC)*(1+aMC*M[ir]/(bMC+M[ir])+
        aNC*TR[ir]/(bRM+TR[ir]))*TC[ir]-delC*
        TC[ir];
```

− Eq. (4.2-3) is programmed.

```
Nt[ir]=DN*Dr(r[ir])*(Nrr[ir]+(1/r[ir])*Nr[ir])+
       DN*Drr(r[ir])*Nr[ir]+
       sN+rN*(1-N[ir]/KN)*(1+aCN*TC[ir]/(bCN+
       TC[ir]))*N[ir]-delN*N[ir];
```

− Eq. (4.2-4) is programmed.

```
TRt[ir]=DTR*Dr(r[ir])*(TRrr[ir]+(1/r[ir])*TRr[ir])+
        DTR*Drr(r[ir])*TRr[ir]+
        rR*(1-TR[ir]/KR)*(1+aMR*M[ir]/(bMR+M[ir]))*
        TR[ir]-delR*TR[ir];
   }
  }
```

The first final } concludes the **for** with $r > 0$. The second final } concludes the stepping through r with index **ir**.

- ODEs (4.2-5,6,7,8) are programmed.

```
#
# Peripheral ODEs
   Mpt= -kM*( Mp- M[nr]);
  TCpt=-kTC*(TCp-TC[nr]);
   Npt= -kN*( Np- N[nr]);
  TRpt=-kTR*(TRp-TR[nr]);
```

ODEs (4.2-5,6,7,8), are added, and with nr=51, give a total of $4 \times 51 + 4 = 4(51) + 4 = 208$ ordinary derivatives in t.

- The 4*nr+4 = 208 derivatives in t are placed in a single vector, ut, for return to lsodes.

```
#
# t derivative vector
  ut=rep(0,4*nr+4);
  for(ir in 1:nr){
    ut[ir]      = Mt[ir];
    ut[ir+nr]   =TCt[ir];
    ut[ir+2*nr]= Nt[ir];
    ut[ir+3*nr]=TRt[ir];
  }
    ut[4*nr+1]= Mpt;
    ut[4*nr+2]=TCpt;
    ut[4*nr+3]= Npt;
    ut[4*nr+4]=TRpt;
```

- The number of calls to pde1a is incremented and returned to the main program by <<-.

```
#
# Increment calls to pde1a
  ncall<<-ncall+1;
```

- The derivative vector of length 208 is returned to lsodes as a list as required by lsodes. c is the R vector utility.

```
#
# Return derivative vector
  return(list(c(ut)));
}
```

The final } concludes pde1a.

(4.1.3) Subordinate routines

Routines Dr,Drr in Listings 4.3, 4.4 for the variable diffusivities follow.

Listing 4.3: Subordinate routine Dr for eq. (4.1-2)

```
Dr=function(r){
#
# Function pde1a computes the variable
# diffusivity
  if((r>=rl)&(r<r1)) {Dr=1;}
  if((r>=r1)&(r<r2)) {Dr=1-0.9/(r2-r1)*(r-r1);}
  if((r>=r2)&(r<=ru)){Dr=0.1;}
#
# Return Dr
  return(c(Dr));
}
```

Listing 4.4: Subordinate routine Drr for eq. (4.1-3)

```
Drr=function(r){
#
# Function pde1a computes the derivative
# of the variable diffusivity
  if((r>=rl)&(r<r1)) {Drr=0;}
  if((r>=r1)&(r<r2)) {Drr=-0.9/(r2-r1);}
  if((r>=r2)&(r<=ru)){Drr=0;}
#
# Return Drr
  return(c(Drr));
}
```

---

r1,r2 are passed directly from the main program to Dr,Drr without special designation (a feature of R).

This completes the discussion of the R coding for eqs. (4.1) through (4.4). Numerical and graphical output is now considered.

(4.1.4)   Numerical, graphical output

Abbreviated numerical output follows in Table 4.1 for ncase=2 (set in the main program of Listing 2.1).

Table 4.1: Abbreviated output for ncase=2

[1] 41

[1] 209

t	r	M(t)	TC(t)	N(t)	TR(t)
0.00	0.00	4.000	464.000	227.000	42.000
0.00	0.10	3.115	361.364	176.788	32.710
0.00	0.20	1.472	170.696	83.509	15.451
0.00	0.30	0.422	48.905	23.926	4.427
0.00	0.40	0.073	8.498	4.158	0.769
0.00	0.50	0.008	0.896	0.438	0.081
0.00	0.60	0.000	0.057	0.028	0.005
0.00	0.70	0.000	0.002	0.001	0.000
0.00	0.80	0.000	0.000	0.000	0.000
0.00	0.90	0.000	0.000	0.000	0.000
0.00	1.00	0.000	0.000	0.000	0.000

t		Mp(t)	TCp(t)	Np(t)	TRp(t)
0.00		0.000	0.000	0.000	0.000

t	r	M(t)	TC(t)	N(t)	TR(t)
100.00	0.00	3.196	469.699	254.231	43.771
100.00	0.10	2.938	442.707	245.250	42.810
100.00	0.20	2.289	350.152	211.775	39.400
100.00	0.30	1.533	197.143	145.451	31.728
100.00	0.40	0.910	67.868	72.035	18.790
100.00	0.50	0.485	13.026	26.613	5.955
100.00	0.60	0.284	1.355	10.175	0.765
100.00	0.70	0.237	0.071	7.065	0.038
100.00	0.80	0.233	0.001	6.835	0.000
100.00	0.90	0.233	0.000	6.832	0.000
100.00	1.00	0.233	0.000	6.828	0.000

t		Mp(t)	TCp(t)	Np(t)	TRp(t)
100.00		0.229	0.000	6.702	0.000

$$\vdots \qquad\qquad\qquad \vdots$$

Output for t = 200,...,900 removed

$$\vdots \qquad\qquad\qquad \vdots$$

(*Continued*)

Table 4.1: (Continued) Abbreviated output for ncase=2

t	r	M(t)	TC(t)	N(t)	TR(t)
1000.00	0.00	5.201	545.017	274.149	47.871
1000.00	0.10	5.201	545.017	274.149	47.871
1000.00	0.20	5.201	545.020	274.150	47.871
1000.00	0.30	5.201	545.027	274.150	47.872
1000.00	0.40	5.202	545.038	274.151	47.873
1000.00	0.50	5.204	545.059	274.152	47.875
1000.00	0.60	5.206	545.098	274.154	47.879
1000.00	0.70	5.212	545.175	274.159	47.886
1000.00	0.80	5.225	545.373	274.171	47.904
1000.00	0.90	5.246	545.665	274.188	47.931
1000.00	1.00	5.255	545.795	274.196	47.943

t	Mp(t)	TCp(t)	Np(t)	TRp(t)
1000.00	5.255	545.799	274.196	47.944

```
ncall =   638
```

We can note the following details about this output.

- 41 output points in t (from nout=41 in the main program of Listing 2.1 as the first dimension of the solution matrix out from lsodes.
- The solution matrix out returned by lsodes has $4(51)+4+1 = 209$ elements as a second dimension. The first element is the value of t. Elements 2 to 205 in out are $M(r,t)$, $T_C(r,t)$, $N(r,t)$, $T_R(r,t)$ for eqs. (4.2-1,2,3,4). Elements 206 to 209 in out are $M_p(t)$, $T_{Cp}(t)$, $N_p(t)$, $T_{Rp}(t)$ for eqs. (4.2-5,6,7,8).
- The solution is displayed for $t = 0, 100, ..., 1000$ and $r = 0, 0.1, ..., 1$ as programmed in Listings 2.1, 3.1 (every fourth value of t and every fifth value of r with nr=51, as discussed previously).
- ICs (4.3) $(t = 0)$ are confirmed. This check is important since if the ICs are not correct, the subsequent solution will also not be correct.
- The solutions vary in r in response to ICs (4.3-1,2,3,4) (Gaussian functions for ncase=2) with the homogeneous Neumann $(r = r_l = 0)$ and Robin $(r = r_u = 1)$ BCs (4.4).
- The computational effort is modest, ncall = 638, so that lsodes efficiently computed a solution to eqs. (4.2) through (4.4).

The graphical output follows in Figures 4.1.

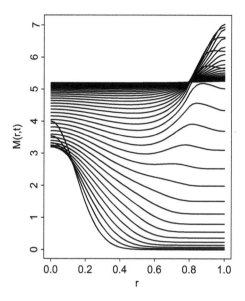

Figure 4.1-1: Numerical solution $M(r,t)$ from eq. (4.2-1), `ncase=2`, `matplot`.

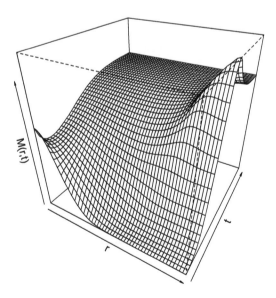

Figure 4.1-2: Numerical solution $M(r,t)$ from eq. (4.2-1), `ncase=2`, `persp`.

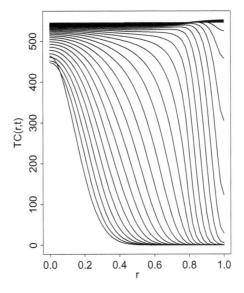

Figure 4.1-3: Numerical solution $T_C(r, t)$ from eq. (4.2-2), `ncase=2`, `matplot`.

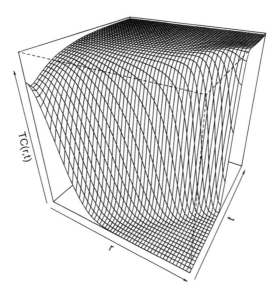

Figure 4.1-4: Numerical solution $T_C(r, t)$ from eq. (4.2-2), `ncase=2`, `persp`.

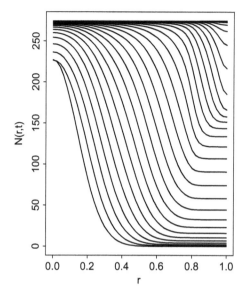

Figure 4.1-5: Numerical solution $N(r,t)$ from eq. (4.2-3), `ncase=2`, `matplot`.

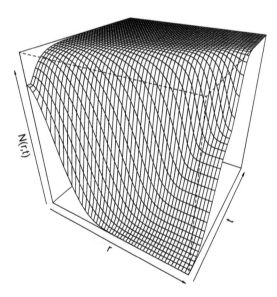

Figure 4.1-6: Numerical solution $N(r,t)$ from eq. (4.2-3), `ncase=2`, `persp`.

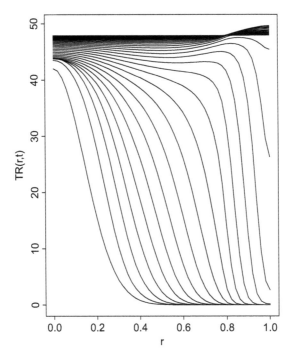

Figure 4.1-7: Numerical solution $T_R(r, t)$ from eq. (4.2-4), `ncase=2`, `matplot`.

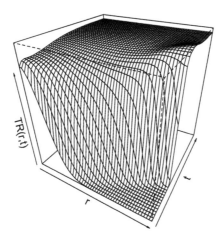

Figure 4.1-8: Numerical solution $T_R(r, t)$ from eq. (4.2-4), `ncase=2`, `persp`.

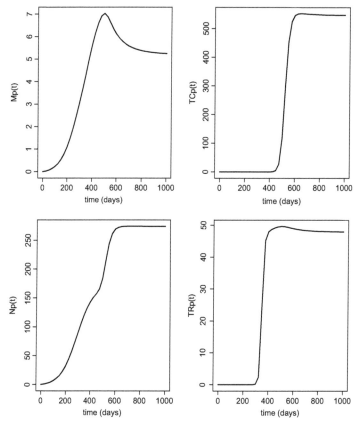

Figure 4.1-9: Numerical solution $M_p(t)$, $T_{Cp}(t)$, $N_p(t)$, $T_{Rp}(t)$ from eqs. (4.2-5,6,7,8), ncase=2.

Figures 4.1 generally confirm the evolution of the numerical solutions from the IC Gaussian functions for the PDEs to the final equilibrium solutions. The effect of the variable diffusivities can be observed by comparing Figures 3.1 (constant diffusivities) and Figures 4.1 (variable diffusivities). Basically, the variable diffusivities delay the response of the peripheral variables, $M_p(t)$, $T_{cp}(t)$, $N_p(t)$, $T_{Rp}(t)$.

(4.2)   Summary and conclusions

The transfer of the four dependent variable components is studied with the ODE/PDE model of Chapter 3, but with diffusivities that vary radially (with respect to r). The MOL implementation is with the main programs of Listings 2.1, 3.1, 4.1, and the ODE/MOL routine of Listing 4.2. Two parameters, r_1, r_2, define the interval in r of a linear variation of the diffusivities. The variation of the diffusivities is defined in function `Dr` of Listing 4.3 and the derivative function `Drr` of Listing 4.4. Generally, the ODE solutions again track the PDE solutions.

A procedure is presented in Chapter 5 for studying the complexity of the solutions in Figures 4.1 based on the examination of the LHS and RHS terms of eqs. (4.2).

5 Detailed Analysis of PDEs in ODE/PDE Model

(5) Introduction

The complexity of the solutions reported in Chapter 4 (see Figures 4.1) suggests further study to gain additional insight into the characteristics of the ODE/PDE model.

(5.1) PDE LHS analysis

In the analysis that follows, the origin of the solution complexity is elucidated by examining the PDE LHS and RHS terms. First, the analysis of the LHS terms is implemented in the following main program and ODE/MOL routine.[1]

(5.1.1) Main program for PDE LHS analysis

The following main program is an extension of the main programs of Listings 2.1, 3.1, and 4.1.

Listing 5.1: Main program for PDE LHSs of eqs. (4.2)

```
#
#  Four ODE/PDE MM model
#
# Access ODE integrator
  library("deSolve");
#
# Access functions for numerical solution
  setwd("f:/multipleMyeloma/chap5");
  source("pde1a.R");
  source("Dr.R");
  source("Drr.R");
  source("dss004.R");
  source("dss044.R");
```

(Continued)

---

[1] PDE - partial differential equation. ODE - ordinary differential equation. LHS - left hand side. RHS - right hand side. MOL - method of lines.

Listing 5.1 (Continued): Main program for PDE LHSs of eqs. (4.2)

```
#
# Select case
#
# ncase-1: PDE Uniform ICs
#
# ncase=2: PDE Gaussian ICs
#
  ncase=2;
#
# Parameters
#
# Eq. (1.1-1)
  sM = 0.001; rM = 0.0175; KM = 10;
  delM = 0.002; aNM = 5; bNM = 150;
  aCM = 5; bCM = 375; aCNM = 8;
  aMM = 0.5; bMM = 3; aRM = 0.5;
  bRM = 25;
#
# Eq. (1.1-2)
  rC =0.013; KC = 800; aMC = 5;
  bMC = 3; aNC = 1; bNC = 150;
  delC = 0.02;
#
# Eq. (1.1-3)
  sN = 0.03; rN = 0.04; KN = 450;
  aCN = 1; bCN= 375; delN = 0.025;
#
# Eq. (1.1-4)
  rR = 0.0831; KR = 80; aMR = 2;
  bMR = 3; delR = 0.0757;
#
# Diffusivities (cm^2/day)
  days=60*60*24;
   DM=1.0e-09*days;
  DTC=1.0e-09*days;
   DN=1.0e-09*days;
  DTR=1.0e-09*days;
   r1=0.4;
   r2=0.8;
```

(Continued)

**Listing 5.1 (Continued): Main program for PDE LHSs
of eqs. (4.2)**

```
#
# Peripheral ODEs
  kM=1; kTC=1;
  kN=1; kTR=1;
#
# Spatial grid
  rl=0; ru=1; nr=51; dr=(ru-rl)/(nr-1);
  r=seq(from=rl,to=ru,by=dr);
#
# Independent variable for ODE integration
  t0=0;tf=1.0e+03;nout=41;dt=(tf-t0)/(nout-1);
  tout=seq(from=t0,to=tf,by=dt);
#
# Initial conditions (t=0)
  u0=rep(0,4*nr+4);
  for(ir in 1:nr){
    if(ncase==1){
      u0[ir]       =4;
      u0[ir+nr]   =464;
      u0[ir+2*nr]=227;
      u0[ir+3*nr]= 42;
    }
    if(ncase==2){
      u0[ir]       =4*exp(-25*r[ir]^2);
      u0[ir+nr]   =464*exp(-25*r[ir]^2);
      u0[ir+2*nr]=227*exp(-25*r[ir]^2);
      u0[ir+3*nr]= 42*exp(-25*r[ir]^2);
    }
  }
  u0[4*nr+1]=0;
  u0[4*nr+2]=0;
  u0[4*nr+3]=0;
  u0[4*nr+4]=0;
  ncall=0;
#
# PDE integration
  nre=1;
  out=lsodes(y=u0,times=tout,func=pde1a,
      sparsetype ="sparseint",rtol=1e-6,
      atol=1e-6,maxord=5);
```

(Continued)

Listing 5.1 (Continued): Main program for PDE LHSs of eqs. (4.2)

```
  nrow(out)
  ncol(out)
#
# Arrays for plotting numerical solution
  M=matrix(0,nrow=nr,ncol=nout);
  TC=matrix(0,nrow=nr,ncol=nout);
  N=matrix(0,nrow=nr,ncol=nout);
  TR=matrix(0,nrow=nr,ncol=nout);
  Mp=rep(0,nout);
  TCp=rep(0,nout);
  Np=rep(0,nout);
  TRp=rep(0,nout);
  for(it in 1:nout){
  for(ir in 1:nr){
     M[ir,it]=out[it,ir+1];
    TC[ir,it]=out[it,ir+nr+1];
     N[ir,it]=out[it,ir+2*nr+1];
    TR[ir,it]=out[it,ir+3*nr+1];
  }
   Mp[it]=out[it,4*nr+2];
  TCp[it]=out[it,4*nr+3];
   Np[it]=out[it,4*nr+4];
  TRp[it]=out[it,4*nr+5];
  }
#
# Display numerical solution
  iv=seq(from=1,to=nout,by=4);
  for(it in iv){
  cat(sprintf("\n\n      t      r        M(t)       TC(t)
             N(t)        TR(t)"));
  iv=seq(from=1,to=nr,by=5);
  for(ir in iv){
    cat(sprintf("\n%6.2f %6.2f %10.3f %10.3f %10.3f %10.3f",
      tout[it],r[ir],M[ir,it],TC[ir,it],N[ir,it],TR[ir,it]));
  }
  cat(sprintf("\n\n      t              Mp(t)      TCp(t)
             Np(t)       TRp(t)"));
  cat(sprintf("\n%6.2f %17.3f %10.3f %10.3f %10.3f",
      tout[it],Mp[it],TCp[it],Np[it],TRp[it]));
  }
```

(Continued)

Listing 5.1 (Continued): Main program for PDE LHSs of eqs. (4.2)

```
#
# Calls to ODE routine
  cat(sprintf("\n\n ncall = %5d\n\n",ncall));
#
# Plot PDE solutions
  par(mfrow=c(1,1));
#
# M(r,t)
#
# 2D
  matplot(r,M,type="l",xlab="r",ylab="M(r,t)",
          lty=1,main="",lwd=2,col="black");
#
# 3D
  persp(r,tout,M,theta=30,phi=30,
        xlim=c(rl,ru),ylim=c(t0,tf),xlab="r",
        ylab="t",zlab="M(r,t)");
#
# TC(r,t)
#
# 2D
  matplot(r,TC,type="l",xlab="r",ylab="TC(r,t)",
          lty=1,main="",lwd=2,col="black");
#
# 3D
  persp(r,tout,TC,theta=30,phi=30,
        xlim=c(rl,ru),ylim=c(t0,tf),xlab="r",
        ylab="t",zlab="TC(r,t)");
#
# N(r,t)
#
# 2D
  matplot(r,N,type="l",xlab="r",ylab="N(r,t)",
          lty=1,main="",lwd=2,col="black");
#
# 3D
  persp(r,tout,N,theta=30,phi=30,
        xlim=c(rl,ru),ylim=c(t0,tf),xlab="r",
        ylab="t",zlab="N(r,t)");
```

(Continued)

Listing 5.1 (Continued): Main program for PDE LHSs of eqs. (4.2)

```
#
# TR(r,t)
#
# 2D
  matplot(r,TR,type="l",xlab="r",ylab="TR(r,t)",
          lty=1,main="",lwd=2,col="black");
#
# 3D
  persp(r,tout,TR,theta=30,phi=30,
        xlim=c(rl,ru),ylim=c(t0,tf),xlab="r",
        ylab="t",zlab="TR(r,t)");
#
# Plot ODE solutions
#
# 2 x 2 matrix of plots
  par(mfrow=c(2,2));
#
# Mp(t)
  plot(tout,Mp,xlab="time (days)",ylab="Mp(t)",
    xlim=c(t0,tf),main="",type="l",lwd=2,
    col="black");
#
# TCp(t)
  plot(tout,TCp,xlab="time (days)",ylab="TCp(t)",
    xlim=c(t0,tf),main="",type="l",lwd=2,
    col="black");
#
# Np(t)
  plot(tout,Np,xlab="time (days)",ylab="Np(t)",
    xlim=c(t0,tf),main="",type="l",lwd=2,
    col="black");
#
# TRp(t)
  plot(tout,TRp,xlab="time (days)",ylab="TRp(t)",
    xlim=c(t0,tf),main="",type="l",lwd=2,
    col="black");
#
# Plot PDE LHS t derivatives
#
```

(Continued)

Listing 5.1 (Continued): Main program for PDE LHSs of eqs. (4.2)

```
# Composite solution vector
  u=matrix(0,nrow=4*nr,ncol=nout);
  for(it in 1:nout){
  for(ir in 1:nr){
    u[ir,it]     = M[ir,it];
    u[ir+nr,it]  =TC[ir,it];
    u[ir+2*nr,it]= N[ir,it];
    u[ir+3*nr,it]=TR[ir,it];
  }
  }
#
# Composite t derivative vector
  ut=matrix(0,nrow=4*nr+4,ncol=nout);
  nre=2;
  for(it in 1:nout){
    ut[,it]=pde1a(tout[it],u[,it],parm);
  }
#
# Composite t derivative vector placed
# in four vectors
   Mt=matrix(0,nrow=nr,ncol=nout);
  TCt=matrix(0,nrow=nr,ncol=nout);
   Nt=matrix(0,nrow=nr,ncol=nout);
  TRt=matrix(0,nrow=nr,ncol=nout);
  for(it in 1:nout){
  for(ir in 1:nr){
     Mt[ir,it]=ut[ir,it];
    TCt[ir,it]=ut[ir+nr,it];
     Nt[ir,it]=ut[ir+2*nr,it];
    TRt[ir,it]=ut[ir+3*nr,it];
  }
  }
#
# Display LHS derivative vectors
  cat(sprintf("\n LHS t derivatives\n"));
#
# Plot PDE LHS derivative vectors
#
# 1 x 1 matrix of plots
  par(mfrow=c(1,1));
```

(Continued)

Listing 5.1 (Continued): Main program for PDE LHSs of eqs. (4.2)

```
#
# Mt(r,t)
#
# 2D
  matplot(r,Mt,type="l",xlab="r",ylab="Mt(r,t)",
          lty=1,main="",lwd=2,col="black");
#
# 3D
  persp(r,tout,Mt,theta=60,phi=45,
        xlim=c(rl,ru),ylim=c(t0,tf),xlab="r",ylab="t",
        zlab="Mt(r,t)");
#
# TCt(r,t)
#
# 2D
  matplot(r,TCt,type="l",xlab="r",ylab="TCt(r,t)",
          lty=1,main="",lwd=2,col="black");
#
# 3D
  persp(r,tout,TCt,theta=60,phi=45,
        xlim=c(rl,ru),ylim=c(t0,tf),xlab="r",ylab="t",
        zlab="TCt(r,t)");
#
# Nt(r,t)
#
# 2D
  matplot(r,Nt,type="l",xlab="r",ylab="Nt(r,t)",
          lty=1,main="",lwd=2,col="black");
#
# 3D
  persp(r,tout, Nt,theta=60,phi=45,
        xlim=c(rl,ru),ylim=c(t0,tf),xlab="r",ylab="t",
        zlab="Nt(r,t)");
#
# TRt(r,t)
#
# 2D
  matplot(r,TRt,type="l",xlab="r",ylab="TRt(r,t)",
          lty=1,main="",lwd=2,col="black");
```

(Continued)

**Listing 5.1 (Continued): Main program for PDE LHSs
of eqs. (4.2)**

```
#
# 3D
  persp(r,tout,TRt,theta=60,phi=45,
        xlim=c(rl,ru),ylim=c(t0,tf),xlab="r",ylab="t",
        zlab="TRt(r,t)");
```

The complete main program of Listing 5.1 is provided so that this concluding example MM application is self-contained, but the following discussion emphasizes just the additional coding (added to Listings 2.1, 3.1, 4.1) for the detailed ODE/PDE analysis.

We can note the following details of Listing 5.1.

- A variable **nre** is added to select the form of the return t derivative vector in the ODE/MOL routine **pde1a** (considered subsequently).

```
#
# PDE integration
  nre=1;
  out=lsodes(y=u0,times=tout,func=pde1a,
      sparsetype ="sparseint",rtol=1e-6,
      atol=1e-6,maxord=5);
  nrow(out)
  ncol(out)
```

- A section of code at the end of the main program calculates and displays (plots) the PDE LHSs (derivative vectors in t). The beginning of this additional code produces a composite vector u of the dependent variables $M(r,t)$, $TC(r,t)$, $N(r,t)$, $TR(r,t)$ of eqs. (4.2-1,2,3,4).

```
#
# Plot PDE LHS t derivatives
#
# Composite solution vector
  u=matrix(0,nrow=4*nr,ncol=nout);
  for(it in 1:nout){
  for(ir in 1:nr){
    u[ir,it]    = M[ir,it];
    u[ir+nr,it]  =TC[ir,it];
```

```
    u[ir+2*nr,it]= N[ir,it];
    u[ir+3*nr,it]=TR[ir,it];
  }
}
```

- The composite derivative vector ut is computed with a call to the ODE/MOL routine pde1a and nre=2.

```
#
# Composite t derivative vector
  ut=matrix(0,nrow=4*nr+4,ncol=nout);
  nre=2;
  for(it in 1:nout){
    ut[,it]=pde1a(tout[it],u[,it],parm);
  }
```

The use of the values nre=1,2 in pde1a is discussed subsequently. pde1a has a 1D vector of dependent variable values as an input, u[,it], and returns a 1D vector of t derivatives, ut[,it]. The set of values of r is specified with a comma, u[,it],ut[,it], for a particular t specified with it.

- The derivatives $\frac{\partial M(r,t)}{\partial t}$, $\frac{\partial T_C(r,t)}{\partial t}$, $\frac{\partial N(r,t)}{\partial t}$, $\frac{\partial T_R(r,t)}{\partial t}$, are taken from ut.

```
#
# Composite t derivative vector placed
# in four vectors
   Mt=matrix(0,nrow=nr,ncol=nout);
  TCt=matrix(0,nrow=nr,ncol=nout);
   Nt=matrix(0,nrow=nr,ncol=nout);
  TRt=matrix(0,nrow=nr,ncol=nout);
  for(it in 1:nout){
  for(ir in 1:nr){
     Mt[ir,it]=ut[ir,it];
    TCt[ir,it]=ut[ir+nr,it];
     Nt[ir,it]=ut[ir+2*nr,it];
    TRt[ir,it]=ut[ir+3*nr,it];
  }
  }
```

- The plotted output is identified.

```
#
# Display LHS derivative vectors
  cat(sprintf("\n LHS t derivatives\n"));
```

- A 2D plot of $\frac{\partial M(r,t)}{\partial t}$ against r and parametrically in t is produced with `matplot`.

```
#
# Plot PDE LHS derivative vectors
#
# 1 x 1 matrix of plots
  par(mfrow=c(1,1));
#
# Mt(r,t)
#
# 2D
  matplot(r,Mt,type="l",xlab="r",ylab="Mt(r,t)",
          lty=1,main="",lwd=2,col="black");
```

`par(mfrow=c(1,1))` specifies one plot on a page.

- A 3D plot of $\frac{\partial M(r,t)}{\partial t}$ against r and t is produced with `persp`.

```
#
# 3D
  persp(r,tout,Mt,theta=60,phi=45,
        xlim=c(rl,ru),ylim=c(t0,tf),xlab="r",ylab="t",
        zlab="Mt(r,t)");
```

- Analogous coding gives 2D and 3D plots of $\frac{\partial T_C(r,t)}{\partial t}$, $\frac{\partial N(r,t)}{\partial t}$, $\frac{\partial T_R(r,t)}{\partial t}$.

```
#
# TCt(r,t)
#
# 2D
  matplot(r,TCt,type="l",xlab="r",ylab="TCt(r,t)",
          lty=1,main="",lwd=2,col="black");
#
# 3D
  persp(r,tout,TCt,theta=60,phi=45,
        xlim=c(rl,ru),ylim=c(t0,tf),xlab="r",ylab="t",
        zlab="TCt(r,t)");
#
# Nt(r,t)
#
# 2D
```

```
    matplot(r,Nt,type="l",xlab="r",ylab="Nt(r,t)",
        lty=1,main="",lwd=2,col="black");
#
# 3D
  persp(r,tout, Nt,theta=60,phi=45,
      xlim=c(rl,ru),ylim=c(t0,tf),xlab="r",ylab="t",
      zlab="Nt(r,t)");
#
# TRt(r,t)
#
# 2D
  matplot(r,TRt,type="l",xlab="r",ylab="TRt(r,t)",
      lty=1,main="",lwd=2,col="black");
#
# 3D
  persp(r,tout,TRt,theta=60,phi=45,
      xlim=c(rl,ru),ylim=c(t0,tf),xlab="r",ylab="t",
      zlab="TRt(r,t)");
```

An important detail is the use of pde1a with nre=2 to calculate the derivative vectors in t.

(5.1.2)   ODE/MOL routine

The ODE/MOL routine pde1a is listed next.

Listing 5.2: ODE/MOL routine for eqs. (4.2)

```
  pde1a=function(t,u,parm){
#
# Function pde1a computes the t derivative
# vector of M(r,t), TR(r,t), N(r,t), TR(r,t),
# Mp(t), TRp(t), Np(t), TRp(t)
#
# One vector to four vectors, four scalars
  M=rep(0,nr);
  TC=rep(0,nr);
  N=rep(0,nr);
  TR=rep(0,nr);
  for(ir in 1:nr){
    M[ir]=u[ir];
```

(Continued)

Listing 5.2 (Continued): ODE/MOL routine for eqs. (4.2)

```
    TC[ir]=u[ir+nr];
     N[ir]=u[ir+2*nr];
    TR[ir]=u[ir+3*nr];
  }
   Mp=u[4*nr+1];
  TCp=u[4*nr+2];
   Np=u[4*nr+3];
  TRp=u[4*nr+4];
#
# Mr,TCr,Nr,TRr
   Mr=dss004(rl,ru,nr, M);
  TCr=dss004(rl,ru,nr,TC);
   Nr=dss004(rl,ru,nr, N);
  TRr=dss004(rl,ru,nr,TR);
#
# BCs
  Mr[1]=0;  Mr[nr]= kM*( Mp- M[nr]);
 TCr[1]=0; TCr[nr]=kTC*(TCp-TC[nr]);
  Nr[1]=0;  Nr[nr]= kN*( Np- N[nr]);
 TRr[1]=0; TRr[nr]=kTR*(TRp-TR[nr]);
#
# Mrr,TCrr,Nrr,TRrr
  nl=2;nu=2;
   Mrr=dss044(rl,ru,nr, M, Mr,nl,nu);
  TCrr=dss044(rl,ru,nr,TC,TCr,nl,nu);
   Nrr=dss044(rl,ru,nr, N, Nr,nl,nu);
  TRrr=dss044(rl,ru,nr,TR,TRr,nl,nu);
#
# PDEs
   Mt=rep(0,nr);
  TCt=rep(0,nr);
   Nt=rep(0,nr);
  TRt=rep(0,nr);
  for(ir in 1:nr){
    if(ir==1){
      Mt[ir]=DM*Dr(r[ir])*2*Mrr[ir]+
             DM*Drr(r[ir])*Mr[ir]+
             sM+rM*(1-M[ir]/KM)*M[ir]-
             delM*(1+(aNM*N[ir]/(bNM+N[ir])+
             aCM*TC[ir]/(bCM+TC[ir])+
             aCNM*N[ir]/(bNM+N[ir])*TC[ir]/(bCM+TC[ir]))*
```

(Continued)

Listing 5.2 (Continued): ODE/MOL routine for eqs. (4.2)

```
                (1-aMM*M[ir]/(bMM+M[ir])-
                aRM*TR[ir]/(bRM+TR[ir])))*M[ir];
    TCt[ir]=DTC*Dr(r[ir])*2*TCrr[ir]+
                DTC*Drr(r[ir])*TCr[ir]+
                rC*(1-TC[ir]/KC)*(1+aMC*M[ir]/(bMC+M[ir])+
                aNC*TR[ir]/(bRM+TR[ir]))*TC[ir]-delC*TC[ir];
    Nt[ir]=DN*Dr(r[ir])*2*Nrr[ir]+
                DN*Drr(r[ir])*Nr[ir]+
                sN+rN*(1-N[ir]/KN)*(1+aCN*TC[ir]/(bCN+TC[ir]))*
                N[ir]-delN*N[ir];
    TRt[ir]=DTR*Dr(r[ir])*2*TRrr[ir]+
                DTR*Drr(r[ir])*TRr[ir]+
                rR*(1-TR[ir]/KR)*(1+aMR*M[ir]/(bMR+M[ir]))*
                TR[ir]-delR*TR[ir];
    }
    if(ir>1){
      Mt[ir]=DM*Dr(r[ir])*(Mrr[ir]+(1/r[ir])*Mr[ir])+
                DM*Drr(r[ir])*Mr[ir]+
                sM+rM*(1-M[ir]/KM)*M[ir]-
                delM*(1+(aNM*N[ir]/(bNM+N[ir])+
                aCM*TC[ir]/(bCM+TC[ir])+
                aCNM*N[ir]/(bNM+N[ir])*TC[ir]/(bCM+TC[ir]))*
                (1-aMM*M[ir]/(bMM+M[ir])-
                aRM*TR[ir]/(bRM+TR[ir])))*M[ir];
    TCt[ir]=DTC*Dr(r[ir])*(TCrr[ir]+(1/r[ir])*TCr[ir])+
                DTC*Drr(r[ir])*TCr[ir]+
                rC*(1-TC[ir]/KC)*(1+aMC*M[ir]/(bMC+M[ir])+
                aNC*TR[ir]/(bRM+TR[ir]))*TC[ir]-delC*TC[ir];
      Nt[ir]=DN*Dr(r[ir])*(Nrr[ir]+(1/r[ir])*Nr[ir])+
                DN*Drr(r[ir])*Nr[ir]+
                sN+rN*(1-N[ir]/KN)*(1+aCN*TC[ir]/(bCN+TC[ir]))*
                N[ir]-delN*N[ir];
    TRt[ir]=DTR*Dr(r[ir])*(TRrr[ir]+(1/r[ir])*TRr[ir])+
                DTR*Drr(r[ir])*TRr[ir]+
                rR*(1-TR[ir]/KR)*(1+aMR*M[ir]/(bMR+M[ir]))*
                TR[ir]-delR*TR[ir];
    }
  }
#
# Peripheral ODEs
   Mpt= -kM*( Mp- M[nr]);
```

(Continued)

Listing 5.2 (Continued): ODE/MOL routine for eqs. (4.2)

```
    TCpt=-kTC*(TCp-TC[nr]);
     Npt= -kN*( Np- N[nr]);
    TRpt=-kTR*(TRp-TR[nr]);
#
# t derivative vector
  ut=rep(0,4*nr+4);
  for(ir in 1:nr){
    ut[ir]     = Mt[ir];
    ut[ir+nr]  =TCt[ir];
    ut[ir+2*nr]= Nt[ir];
    ut[ir+3*nr]=TRt[ir];
  }
    ut[4*nr+1]= Mpt;
    ut[4*nr+2]=TCpt;
    ut[4*nr+3]= Npt;
    ut[4*nr+4]=TRpt;
#
# Increment calls to pde1a
  ncall<<-ncall+1;
#
# Return derivative vector
# as a list
  if(nre==1){
    return(list(c(ut)));}
#
# Return derivative vector
# as a numerical vector
  if(nre==2){
    return(c(ut));}
}
```

---

pde1a of Listing 5.2 is the same as **pde1a** of Listing 4.2 except for the addition of coding at the end to specify the form of the returned t derivative vector using nre.

```
#
# Return derivative vector
# as a list
  if(nre==1){
    return(list(c(ut)));}
#
```

```
# Return derivative vector
# as a numerical vector
  if(nre==2){
    return(c(ut));}
}
```

For **nre=1**, the derivative vector **ut** is returned as a **list** to **lsodes** called in the main program of Listing 5.1, as required by **lsodes**. For **nre=2**, the derivative vector **ut** is returned as a numerical vector (with c) to facilitate the plotting in the main program. The final } concludes **pde1a**.

This concludes the programming for the PDE derivatives in t. The output follows.

(5.1.3)   Numerical, graphical output

The numerical ouput from Listings 5.1, 5.2 follows.

Table 5.1: Numerical output from Listings 5.1, 5.2

[1] 41

[1] 209

t	r	M(t)	TC(t)	N(t)	TR(t)
0.00	0.00	4.000	464.000	227.000	42.000
0.00	0.10	3.115	361.364	176.788	32.710
0.00	0.20	1.472	170.696	83.509	15.451
0.00	0.30	0.422	48.905	23.926	4.427
0.00	0.40	0.073	8.498	4.158	0.769
0.00	0.50	0.008	0.896	0.438	0.081
0.00	0.60	0.000	0.057	0.028	0.005
0.00	0.70	0.000	0.002	0.001	0.000
0.00	0.80	0.000	0.000	0.000	0.000
0.00	0.90	0.000	0.000	0.000	0.000
0.00	1.00	0.000	0.000	0.000	0.000

t		Mp(t)	TCp(t)	Np(t)	TRp(t)
0.00		0.000	0.000	0.000	0.000

.
.
.

Output for t = 100, 200, ..., 900 removed

.
.
.

| t | r | M(t) | TC(t) | N(t) | TR(t) |

(Continued)

Table 5.1: (Continued) Numerical output from Listings 5.1, 5.2

1000.00	0.00	5.201	545.017	274.149	47.871
1000.00	0.10	5.201	545.017	274.149	47.871
1000.00	0.20	5.201	545.020	274.150	47.871
1000.00	0.30	5.201	545.027	274.150	47.872
1000.00	0.40	5.202	545.038	274.151	47.873
1000.00	0.50	5.204	545.059	274.152	47.875
1000.00	0.60	5.206	545.098	274.154	47.879
1000.00	0.70	5.212	545.175	274.159	47.886
1000.00	0.80	5.225	545.373	274.171	47.904
1000.00	0.90	5.246	545.665	274.188	47.931
1000.00	1.00	5.255	545.795	274.196	47.943

t	Mp(t)	TCp(t)	Np(t)	TRp(t)
1000.00	5.255	545.799	274.196	47.944

```
ncall =    638

LHS t derivatives
```

The graphical output is in Figures 5.1

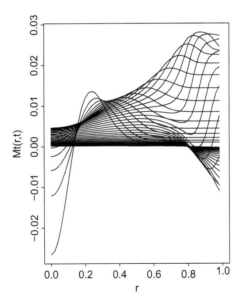

Figure 5.1-1: $\dfrac{\partial M(r,t)}{\partial t}$ from eq. (4.2-1), ncase=2, matplot.

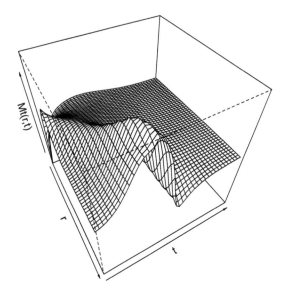

Figure 5.1-2: $\dfrac{\partial M(r,t)}{\partial t}$ from eq. (4.2-1), ncase=2, persp.

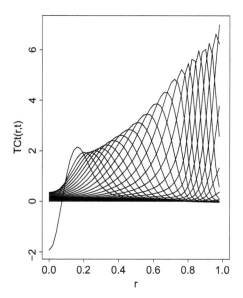

Figure 5.1-3: $\dfrac{\partial T_C(r,t)}{\partial t}$ from eq. (4.2-2), ncase=2, matplot.

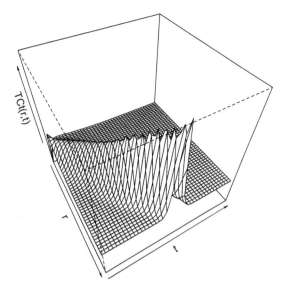

Figure 5.1-4: $\dfrac{\partial T_C(r,t)}{\partial t}$ from eq. (4.2-2), `ncase=2`, `persp`.

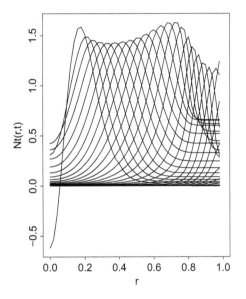

Figure 5.1-5: $\dfrac{\partial N(r,t)}{\partial t}$ from eq. (4.2-3), `ncase=2`, `matplot`.

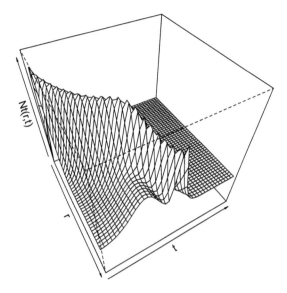

Figure 5.1-6: $\dfrac{\partial N(r,t)}{\partial t}$ from eq. (4.2-3), `ncase=2`, `persp`.

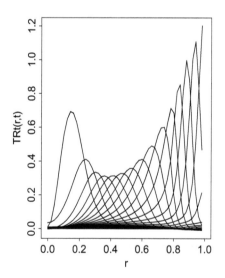

Figure 5.1-7: $\dfrac{\partial T_R(r,t)}{\partial t}$ from eq. (4.2-4), `ncase=2`, `matplot`.

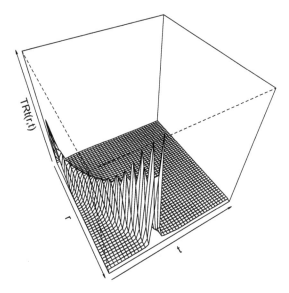

Figure 5.1-8: $\dfrac{\partial T_R(r,t)}{\partial t}$ from eq. (4.2-4), `ncase=2`, `persp`.

Figures 5.1 indicate that the derivatives in t approach zero for the equilibrium (steady state) solutions.

(5.2)   PDE RHS analysis

The complexity of the solutions in Figures 5.1 suggests further analysis of the PDEs, eqs. (4.2-1,2,3,4). Specifically, the RHS terms of the PDEs can be computed and displayed. To illustrate this procedure, the RHS terms of the PDE for $N(r,t)$, eq. (4.2-3), are studied next.

(5.2.1)   Main program for *N(r,t)* PDE RHS analysis

The addition to the end of the main program of Listing 5.1 follows.

Listing 5.3: Addition to Main program of Listing 5.1 for eq. (4.2-3) RHS analysis

```
#
# Plot RHS terms in N PDE
#
# Radial transport (term1)
  Nr=matrix(0,nrow=nr,ncol=nout);
  Nrr=matrix(0,nrow=nr,ncol=nout);
  nl=2;nu=2;
  term1=matrix(0,nrow=nr,ncol=nout);
  for(it in 1:nout){
    Nr[,it]=dss004(rl,ru,nr,N[,it]);
    Nr[1,it]=0;Nr[nr,it]=kN*(Np[it]-N[nr,it]);
   Nrr[,it]=dss044(rl,ru,nr,N[,it],Nr[,it],nl,nu);
   for(ir in 1:nr){
     if(ir==1){
       term1[ir,it]=DN*Dr(r[ir])*2*Nrr[ir,it]+
                    DN*Drr(r[ir])*Nr[ir,it];}
     if(ir>1){
       term1[ir,it]=DN*Dr(r[ir])*(Nrr[ir,it]+(1/r[ir])*
                    Nr[ir,it])+DN*Drr(r[ir])*Nr[ir,it];}
   }
   }
#
# 2D
  matplot(r,term1,type="l",xlab="r",ylab="term1",
          lty=1,main="",lwd=2,col="black");
#
# Volumetric generation (term2)
  term2=matrix(0,nrow=nr,ncol=nout);
  for(it in 1:nout){
  for(ir in 1:nr){
    term2[ir,it]=sN+rN*(1-N[ir,it]/KN)*
      (1+aCN*TC[ir,it]/(bCN+TC[ir,it]))*N[ir,it];
  }
  }
```

(Continued)

```
Listing 5.3 (Continued): Addition to Main program of Listing
                5.1 for eq. (4.2-3) RHS analysis

#
# 2D
  matplot(r,term2,type="l",xlab="r",ylab="term2",
          lty=1,main="",lwd=2,col="black");
#
# Volumetric depletion (term3)
  term3=matrix(0,nrow=nr,ncol=nout);
  for(it in 1:nout){
  for(ir in 1:nr){
    term3[ir,it]=-delN*N[ir,it];
  }
  }
#
# 2D
  matplot(r,term3,type="l",xlab="r",ylab="term3",
          lty=1,main="",lwd=2,col="black");
```

We can note the following details about this coding.

- The radial transport term in eq. (4.2-1), $D_N D(r) \left(\frac{\partial^2 N}{\partial r^2} + \frac{1}{r} \frac{\partial N}{\partial r} \right) + D_N \frac{dD(r)}{dr} \frac{\partial N}{\partial r}$, denoted as term1, is computed as a function of r and t.

```
#
# Plot RHS terms in N PDE
#
# Radial transport (term1)
    Nr=matrix(0,nrow=nr,ncol=nout);
    Nrr=matrix(0,nrow=nr,ncol=nout);
    nl=2;nu=2;
    term1=matrix(0,nrow=nr,ncol=nout);
    for(it in 1:nout){
      Nr[,it]=dss004(rl,ru,nr,N[,it]);
      Nr[1,it]=0;Nr[nr,it]=kN*(Np[it]-N[nr,it]);
      Nrr[,it]=dss044(rl,ru,nr,N[,it],Nr[,it],nl,nu);
      for(ir in 1:nr){
        if(ir==1){
          term1[ir,it]=
          DN*Dr(r[ir])*2*Nrr[ir,it]+
          DN*Drr(r[ir])*Nr[ir,it];}
```

```
    if(ir>1){
      term1[ir,it]=
      DN*Dr(r[ir])*(Nrr[ir,it]+(1/r[ir])*Nr[ir,it])+
      DN*Drr(r[ir])*Nr[ir,it];}
  }
  }
```

We can note the following details about this coding.

- Two `fors` are used to step through t and r.
- `dss004` has a 1D vector of dependent variable values as an input, `N[,it]`, and returns a 1D vector of first order r derivatives, `Nr[,it]`. The set of values of r is specified with a comma, `N[,it]`, `Nr[,it]`, for a particular t specified with `it`.
- Similarly, `dss044` has two 1D vectors, `N[,it]` and `Nr[,it]`, as inputs, and returns a 1D vector of second order r derivatives, `Nrr[,it]`. BCs (4.4-5,6) are included in the calculation of `Nrr` with Neumann BCs specified with `nl=nu=2`.
- The radial group

$$D_N D(r) \left(\frac{\partial^2 N}{\partial r^2} + \frac{1}{r} \frac{\partial N}{\partial r} \right) + D_N \frac{dD(r)}{dr} \frac{\partial N}{\partial r} \qquad (5.1\text{-}1)$$

is programmed for $r = 0$ (which includes the regularization of the indeterminant term

$$\frac{1}{r} \frac{\partial N}{\partial r} \Big|_{r=0} = \frac{\partial^2 N}{\partial r^2}$$

```
    if(ir==1){
      term1[ir,it]=
      DN*Dr(r[ir])*2*Nrr[ir,it]+
      DN*Drr(r[ir])*Nr[ir,it];}
```

- The radial group (5.1-1) is programmed for $r > 0$.

```
    if(ir>1){
      term1[ir,it]=
      DN*Dr(r[ir])*(Nrr[ir,it]+(1/r[ir])*Nr[ir,it])+
      DN*Drr(r[ir])*Nr[ir,it];}
```

- The final `}` concludes the `for` in r with index `ir`.
- The radial group (5.1-1) is plotted in 2D with `matplot`.

```
#
# 2D
  matplot(r,term1,type="l",xlab="r",ylab="term1",
          lty=1,main="",lwd=2,col="black");
```

- The volumetric generation rate for $N(r,t)$ (**term2**)

$$+s_N + r_N \left(1 - \frac{N}{K_N}\right)\left(1 + \frac{a_{CN}T_C}{b_{CN} + T_C}\right)N \qquad (5.1\text{-}2)$$

is computed as a function of r and t, then plotted.

```
#
# Volumetric generation (term2)
  term2=matrix(0,nrow=nr,ncol=nout);
  for(it in 1:nout){
  for(ir in 1:nr){
    term2[ir,it]=sN+rN*(1-N[ir,it]/KN)*
      (1+aCN*TC[ir,it]/(bCN+TC[ir,it]))*N[ir,it];
  }
  }
#
# 2D
  matplot(r,term2,type="l",xlab="r",ylab="term2",
          lty=1,main="",lwd=2,col="black");
```

- The volumetric depletion rate for $N(r,t)$ (**term3**)

$$-\delta_N N \qquad (5.1\text{-}3)$$

is computed as a function of r and t, then plotted.

```
#
# Volumetric depletion (term3)
  term3=matrix(0,nrow=nr,ncol=nout);
  for(it in 1:nout){
  for(ir in 1:nr){
    term3[ir,it]=-delN*N[ir,it];
  }
  }
#
# 2D
  matplot(r,term3,type="l",xlab="r",ylab="term3",
          lty=1,main="",lwd=2,col="black");
```

This completes the programming of the RHS terms of eq. (4.2-3) for $N(r,t)$. pde1a from Listing 5.2 is used again.

(5.2.2) Graphical output

The graphical output follows (only the additional plots for `term1`,`term2`, `term3` are indicated since the numerical output is the same as from Listing 5.1 and the other plots are in Figures 4.1 and 5.1).

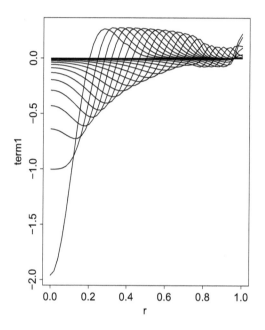

Figure 5.2-1: `term1` from eq. (4.2-3), `ncase=2`, `matplot`.

Figure 5.2-1 indicates that **term1** approaches zero for the contribution to the equilibrium (steady state) solution.

Figure 5.2-2 indicates that **term2** approaches ≈ 6.8 for the contribution to the equilibrium (steady state) solution.

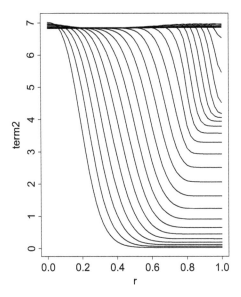

Figure 5.2-2: term2 from eq. (4.2-3), ncase=2, matplot.

Figure 5.2-3 indicates that **term3** approaches ≈ -6.8 for the contribution to the equilibrium (steady state) solution.

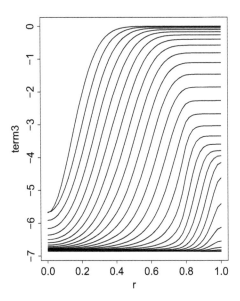

Figure 5.2-3: term3 from eq. (4.2-3), ncase=2, matplot.

In summary, at steady state, $\dfrac{\partial N}{\partial t} = $ term1+term2+term3 $= 0$ as indicated in Figure 5.1-5.

The complexity of term1 in Figure 5.2-1 suggests further study by examining the terms within term1. For example, the two radial terms in term (5.1-1)

$$D_N D(r) \left(\frac{\partial^2 N}{\partial r^2} + \frac{1}{r} \frac{\partial N}{\partial r} \right) \tag{5.1-4}$$

$$+D_N \frac{dD(r)}{dr} \frac{\partial N}{\partial r} \tag{5.1-5}$$

can be compared to determine the effect of the variable diffusivity (function of r). This is done with the following code added to Listings 5.1 and 5.2.

Listing 5.4: Analysis of the radial diffusion in eq. (4.2-3) (term1)

```
#
# Plot terms in term1 of the N PDE
#
  term11=matrix(0,nrow=nr,ncol=nout);
  term12=matrix(0,nrow=nr,ncol=nout);
  for(it in 1:nout){
  for(ir in 1:nr){
    if(ir==1){
      term11[ir,it]=DN*Dr(r[ir])*2*Nrr[ir,it];
      term12[ir,it]=DN*Drr(r[ir])*Nr[ir,it];}
    if(ir>1){
      term11[ir,it]=DN*Dr(r[ir])*(Nrr[ir,it]+(1/r[ir])*
                    Nr[ir,it]);
      term12[it,it]=DN*Drr(r[ir])*Nr[ir,it];}
  }
  }
#
# 2D
#
# term11
  matplot(r,term11,type="l",xlab="r",ylab="term11",
          lty=1,main="",lwd=2,col="black");
#
# term12
  matplot(r,term12,type="l",xlab="r",ylab="term12",
          lty=1,main="",lwd=2,col="black");
```

We can note the following details of the additional code of Listing 5.4.

- Term (5.1-4) is programmed as `term11`.

```
if(ir==1){
  term11[ir,it]=
  DN*Dr(r[ir])*2*Nrr[ir,it];
if(ir>1){
  term11[ir,it]=
  DN*Dr(r[ir])*(Nrr[ir,it]+(1/r[ir])*Nr[ir,it]);
```

- Term (5.1-5) is programmed as `term12`.

```
term12[ir,it]=
DN*Drr(r[ir])*Nr[ir,it];}
```

- `term11,term12` are plotted.

```
#
# 2D
#
# term11
  matplot(r,term11,type="l",xlab="r",ylab="term11",
          lty=1,main="",lwd=2,col="black");
#
# term12
  matplot(r,term12,type="l",xlab="r",ylab="term12",
          lty=1,main="",lwd=2,col="black");
```

Figures 5.3 are the grapical output from Listing 5.4.

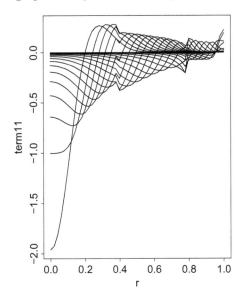

Figure 5.3-1: Term (5.1-4) (`term11`), ncase=2, `matplot`.

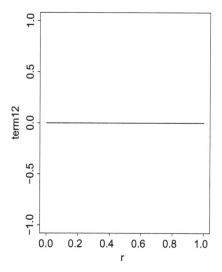

Figure 5.3-2: Term $(5.1\text{-}5)$ $(\texttt{term12})$, $\texttt{ncase=2}$, $\texttt{matplot}$.

Term $(5.1\text{-}5)$ (Figure 5.3-2) is negligible compared to term $(5.1\text{-}4)$ (Figure 5.3-1) (note the vertical scales of Figures 5.3). The reason for this is elucidated with the following remaining code.

Listing 5.5: Analysis of the variable diffusion term in eq. (4.2-3) (term12)

```
#
# Plot factors in term12 of the N PDE
#
  term121=matrix(0,nrow=nr,ncol=nout);
  term122=matrix(0,nrow=nr,ncol=nout);
  for(it in 1:nout){
  for(ir in 1:nr){
     term121[ir,it]=DN*Drr(r[ir]);
     term122[ir,it]=Nr[ir,it];
  }
  }
```

(Continued)

Listing 5.5 (Continued): Analysis of the variable diffusion term in eq. (4.2-3) (term12)

```
#
# 2D
#
# term121
  matplot(r,term121,type="l",xlab="r",ylab="term121",
          lty=1,main="",lwd=2,col="black",
          ylim=c(-2.0e-04,2.0e-04));
  cat(sprintf("\n DN*Drr = %6.3e\n",1.0e-09*60*60*24*
              (-0.9/(r2-r1))));
#
# term122
  matplot(r,term122,type="l",xlab="r",ylab="term122",
          lty=1,main="",lwd=2,col="black");
```

We can note the following details of the additional code for

$$D_N \frac{dD(r)}{dr} \frac{\partial N}{\partial r} \tag{5.1-6}$$

from the radial group of eq. (4.2-3).

- **term121** is the factor $D_N \frac{dD(r)}{dr}$ in term (5.1-6).

  ```
  term121[ir,it]=DN*Drr(r[ir]);
  ```

- **term122** is the factor $\frac{\partial N}{\partial r}$ in term (5.1-6).

  ```
  term122[ir,it]=Nr[ir,it];
  ```

- The graphical output in Figures 5.4 indicates **term121**$= D_N \frac{dD(r)}{dr} = (1.0 \times 10^{-9})(60)(60)(24)(-0.9)/(0.8-0.4) = -0.0001944$ is negligible compared to **term122** $= \frac{\partial N}{\partial r}$ which makes term (5.1-5) negligible compared to (5.1-4).

The graphical output, Figures 5.4, follows.

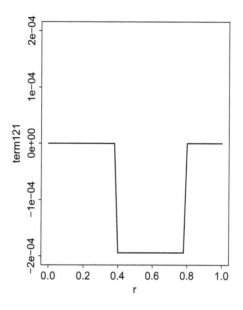

Figure 5.4-1: `term121, ncase=2, matplot.`

`term121` has the expected form from eq. (4.1-3) and the minimum value -0.0001944.

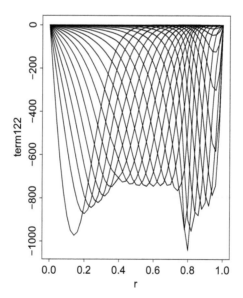

Figure 5.4-2: `term122, ncase=2, matplot.`

Note that `term122` is multiplied (attenuated) by `term121` in forming term (5.1-6).

(5.3) Summary and conclusion

The preceding discussion is intended to illustrate how the detailed analysis of the LHS and RHS terms of a PDE can be refined to the extent that the contribution of each term can be observed and evaluated. This detailed information can then be used to formulate, evaluate and modify a PDE model or an ODE/PDE model. This methodology for a detailed PDE analysis is applied to eq. (4.2-3) of the MM model of eqs. (4.2) to explain the spatiotemporal distribution of $N(r, t)$, one of the four dependent variables of Table 1.1.

Appendix A1: Functions dss004, dss044

(A1.1) Function dss004

A listing of function dss004 follows.

```
  dss004=function(xl,xu,n,u) {
#
# An extensive set of documentation comments detailing
# the derivation of the following fourth order finite
# differences (FDs) is not given here to conserve
# space.  The derivation is detailed in Schiesser,
# W. E., The Numerical Method of Lines Integration
# of Partial Differential Equations, Academic Press,
# San Diego, 1991.
#
# Preallocate arrays
  ux=rep(0,n);
#
# Grid spacing
  dx=(xu-xl)/(n-1);
#
# 1/(12*dx) for subsequent use
  r12dx=1/(12*dx);
#
# ux vector
#
# Boundaries (x=xl,x=xu)
  ux[1]=r12dx*(-25*u[1]+48*u[ 2]-36*u[ 3]+16*u[ 4]-3*u[ 5]);
  ux[n]=r12dx*( 25*u[n]-48*u[n-1]+36*u[n-2]-16*u[n-3]+3*u[n-4]);
#
# dx in from boundaries (x=xl+dx,x=xu-dx)
  ux[ 2]=r12dx*(-3*u[1]-10*u[ 2]+18*u[ 3]-6*u[ 4]+u[ 5]);
  ux[n-1]=r12dx*( 3*u[n]+10*u[n-1]-18*u[n-2]+6*u[n-3]-u[n-4]);
```
(Continued)

```
#
# Interior points (x=xl+2*dx,...,x=xu-2*dx)
  for(i in 3:(n-2))ux[i]=r12dx*(-u[i+2]+8*u[i+1]-8*u[i-1]+
                                u[i-2]);
#
# All points concluded (x=xl,...,x=xu)
  return(c(ux));
}
```

The input arguments are

> xl   lower boundary value of x
>
> xu   upper boundary value of x
>
> n   number of points in the grid in x,
>   including the end points
>
> u   dependent variable to be differentiated,
>   an n-vector

The output, ux, is an n-vector of numerical values of the first derivative of u.

The finite difference (FD) approximations are a weighted sum of the dependent variable values. For example, at point i

```
for(i in 3:(n-2))ux[i]=r12dx*(-u[i+2]+8*u[i+1]-8*u[i-1]+u[i-2]);
```

The weighting coefficients are -1, 8, 0, -8, 1 at points i-2, i-1, i, i+1, i+2, respectievly. These weighting coefficients are antisymmetric (opposite sign) around the center point i because the computed first derivative is of odd order. If the derivative is of even order, the weighting coefficients would be symmetric (same sign) around the center point (as in dss044 that follows).

For i=1. the dependent variable at points i=1,2,3,4,5 is used in the FD approximation for ux[1] to remain within the x domain (fictitious points outside the x domain are not used).

```
ux[1]=r12dx*(-25*u[1]+48*u[2]-36*u[3]+16*u[4]-3*u[5]);
```

Similarly, for i=2, points i=1,2,3,4,5 are used in the FD approximation for ux[2] to remain within the x domain (fictitious points outside the x domain are avoided).

```
ux[2]=r12dx*(-3*u[1]-10*u[2]+18*u[3]-6*u[4]+u[5]);
```

At the right boundary $x = x_u$, points at i=n,n-1,n-2,n-3,n-4 are used for
ux[n],ux[n-1] to avoid points outside the x domain.

In all cases, the FD approximations are fourth order correct in x.

(A1.2) Function dss044

A listing of function dss044 follows.

```
dss044=function(xl,xu,n,u,ux,nl,nu) {
#
# The derivation of the finite difference
# approximations for a second derivative are
# in Schiesser, W. E., The Numerical Method
# of Lines Integration of Partial Differential
# Equations, Academic Press, San Diego, 1991.
#
# Preallocate arrays
  uxx=rep(0,n);
#
# Grid spacing
  dx=(xu-xl)/(n-1);
#
# 1/(12*dx**2) for subsequent use
  r12dxs=1/(12*dx^2);
#
# uxx vector
#
# Boundaries (x=xl,x=xu)
  if(nl==1)
    uxx[1]=r12dxs*
            (45*u[  1]-154*u[  2]+214*u[  3]-
            156*u[  4] +61*u[  5] -10*u[  6]);
  if(nu==1)
    uxx[n]=r12dxs*
            (45*u[  n]-154*u[n-1]+214*u[n-2]-
            156*u[n-3] +61*u[n-4] -10*u[n-5]);
  if(nl==2)
    uxx[1]=r12dxs*
            (-415/6*u[  1] +96*u[  2]-36*u[  3]+
            32/3*u[  4]-3/2*u[  5]-50*ux[1]*dx);
```
                                              (Continued)

```
   if(nu==2)
     uxx[n]=r12dxs*
            (-415/6*u[  n] +96*u[n-1]-36*u[n-2]+
              32/3*u[n-3]-3/2*u[n-4]+50*ux[n]*dx);
#
# dx in from boundaries (x=xl+dx,x=xu-dx)
     uxx[  2]=r12dxs*
            (10*u[  1]-15*u[  2]-4*u[  3]+
             14*u[  4]- 6*u[  5]  +u[  6]);
     uxx[n-1]=r12dxs*
            (10*u[  n]-15*u[n-1]-4*u[n-2]+
             14*u[n-3]- 6*u[n-4]  +u[n-5]);
#
# Remaining interior points (x=xl+2*dx,...,
# x=xu-2*dx)
   for(i in 3:(n-2))
     uxx[i]=r12dxs*
            (-u[i-2]+16*u[i-1]-30*u[i]+
            16*u[i+1]    -u[i+2]);
#
# All points concluded (x=xl,...,x=xu)
   return(c(uxx));
}
```

The input arguments are

xl	lower boundary value of x
xu	upper boundary value of x
n	number of points in the grid in x, including the end points
u	dependent variable to be differentiated, an n-vector
ux	first derivative of u with boundary condition (BC) values, an n-vector

nl   type of boundary condition at x=xl
     1: Dirichlet BC
     2: Neumann BC

nu   type of boundary condition at x=xu
     1: Dirichlet BC
     2: Neumann BC

The output, uxx, is an *n*-vector of numerical values of the second derivative of u.

The finite difference (FD) approximations are a weighted sum of the dependent variable values. For example, at point i

```
for(i in 3:(n-2))
  uxx[i]=r12dxs*
        (-u[i-2]+16*u[i-1]-30*u[i]+
        16*u[i+1]   -u[i+2]);
```

The weighting coefficients are -1, 16, -30, 16, -1 at points i-2, i-1, i, i+1, i+2, respectievly. These weighting coefficients are symmetric around the center point i because the computed second derivative is of even order. If the derivative is of odd order, the weighting coefficients would be antisymmetric (opposite sign) around the center point.

For nl=2 and/or nu=2 the boundary values of the first derivative are included in the FD approximation for the second derivative, uxx. For example, at x=xl (with nl=2),

```
if(nl==2)
  uxx[1]=r12dxs*
        (-415/6*u[  1] +96*u[  2]-36*u[  3]+
        32/3*u[  4]-3/2*u[  5]-50*ux[1]*dx);
```

In computing the second derivative at the left boundary, uxx[1], the first derivative at the left boundary is included, that is, ux[1]. In this way, a Neumann BC is accommodated (ux[1] is included in the input argument ux).

For nl=1, only values of the dependent variable (and not the first derivative) are included in the weighted sum.

```
if(nl==1)
  uxx[1]=r12dxs*
        (45*u[  1]-154*u[  2]+214*u[  3]-
        156*u[  4] +61*u[  5] -10*u[  6]);
```

The dependent variable at points i=1,2,3,4,5,6 is used in the FD approximation for uxx[1] to remain within the x domain (fictitious points outside the x domain are not used).

Six points are used rather than five (as in the centered approximation for uxx[i]) since the FD applies at the left boundary and is not centered (around i). Six points provide a fourth order FD approximation which is the same order as the FDs at the interior points in x.

Similar considerations apply at the upper boundary value of x with nu=1,2.

Robin boundary conditions can also be accommodated with nl=2, nu=2. In all three cases, Dirichlet, Neumann and Robin, the boundary conditions can be linear and/or nonlinear.

Additional details concerning dss004, dss044 are available from [1].

Reference

1. Griffiths, G.W., and W.E. Schiesser (2012), *Traveling Wave Analysis of Partial Differential Equations*, Elsevier/Academic Press, Boston, MA.

Index

For Product Safety Concerns and Information please contact our EU
representative GPSR@taylorandfrancis.com
Taylor & Francis Verlag GmbH, Kaufingerstraße 24, 80331 München, Germany

www.ingramcontent.com/pod-product-compliance
Ingram Content Group UK Ltd.
Pitfield, Milton Keynes, MK11 3LW, UK
UKHW021122180425
457613UK00005B/192